Julian Chitta

TATTOOS

AND THEIR SIGNIFICANCE

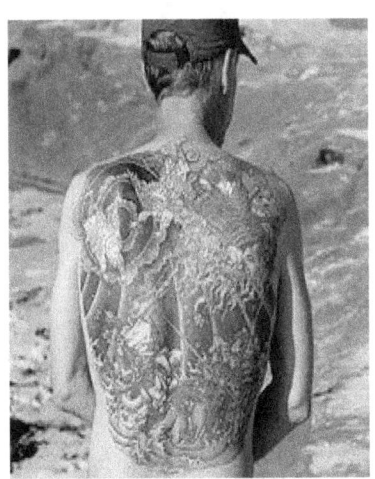

Copyright © 2018 by Julian Chitta. All rights reserved

Editorial & proofing services provided by

Anchor Publishing

P O Box 0731

Kingsland, TX 78639-0731

United States of America

Note: The author of this booklet is the recipient of the Albert Nelson Marquis 2017 Lifetime Achievement Award for Literary Excellence.

CONTENTS

Introduction	5
What is a Tattoo?	8
Why Tattoos	14
Jailbirds and Prison Gangs	19
White Prison Gangs	22
Black Prison Gangs	25
Hispanic Prison Gangs	27
Russian Criminal Gangs	34
Oriental Criminal Gangs	37
Hidden Meaning of Tattoos	43
Poor-Judgment Tattoos	51
Religious Tattoos	57
The Muslim Brotherhood	67
Political Gangs	76
Tattoo Removal	77
Epilogue	83
Bibliography	89

INTRODUCTION

The practice of tattooing goes back millennia. Some of the mummies, over 3,000 years old, found in the Egyptian pyramids, had complex tattoos.

All types of primitive cultures used tattooing as a way to assert a superior social status, or, simply, for aesthetic satisfaction. From the jungles of Africa, to the remote islands of the Pacific, men and women embellished their dermis with tattoos.

No one shall be surprised that modern people use the same procedures to inject inks under their skin. Of course, the techniques, and the graphic realization is much more advanced. If the primitive man and woman used tattooing primarily for social identification and perceived beauty, our contemporaries practice the art of tattooing for additional scopes.

People today use tattoos to assert their social position, to affirm affiliation to certain groups – in many cases to criminal gangs – to advertise their likes and dislikes in various areas, from professions and politics, to hobbies.

The first contact Europeans had with tattooed people, occurred in the 18th century during the era of the great discoveries on exploration voyages, and on colonization campaigns. When the first English and Portuguese sailors met the Pacific populations who maintained a tattoo culture, they learned fast, how to do that, and imported the tattooing procedures into Europe.

At first, the general public looked in disbelief at the tattooed arms of the sailors who circumnavigated the globe, and some enterprising souls took notice seeking information about how to duplicate that.

During the 17th and the 18th centuries tattooing became a form of art that only well-to-do people could afford it.

Shortly, after the tattooing lost its novelty, people sporting them were looked upon as atavisms remained entrenched in the collective psyche for over two centuries. Today, over 50% of population has a dim view of the tattoos, associating them with negative social attributes. It is no secret that most all prison gangs practice tattooing as means of displaying gang affiliation or pride. Practically, all parts of the human body were subject to tattooing, including the genitals. Displaying some of those tattoos in public is considered extremely offensive. Several sociology studies reveal that there is a certain group, between 15 – 30 years of age, with a favorable opinion about tattooing. Some 25% of male adults have tattoos, while only some 20 % of females do. Tattoos are much more prevalent in urban areas, because in the rural area the religious precepts are respected by more people. According to Biblical concepts the human body is a temple dedicated to God, and the tattoos are tantamount to graffiti on that temple, thus an unpardonable sin. Jews and Catholics discourage firmly the practice of tattooing.

The common belief, that less educated people have more tattoos, can be verified statistically. There is no common denominator among the various styles of graphic designs of tattoos. Various ethnic groups prefer certain colors, while the lettering has no specific meaning. English, German and Scandinavian people prefer high Gothic letters. Hispanics and other Europeans like cursive Latin letters.

Russians use Slavic Cyrillic letters, in their tattoos, while Greek and Arabs use their respective alphabets. Normally, it takes an experienced specialist to decode and to interpret the full significance of certain tattoos, a field in which the world's police departments, such like Interpol, and the FBI, do an outstanding job.

Tattoos basically advertise a person's state of mind, vis-à-vis the owner's adherence to a specific social group, most of the time based on anti-social attitudes.

In some countries police specialists collect and catalog tattoo images during the booking of criminal elements, when they also harvest DNA samples. Getting to be familiar with tattoo imagery is today an integral part of the war against organized crime gangs, either in, or out of jails.

Sorting out the types of persons sporting tattoos, leads to the discovery of gang cultures, centered on specific illegal activities, such as drug manufacturing or smuggling, gambling, human trafficking, child prostitution, loansharking, contract killing, and counterfeiting tangible or intellectual property items. Organized in gangs of untold sizes, they maintain a severe discipline, guarding their sources of income by extreme measures, which include murder.

The practice of tattooing is dictated by ancient customs, most often replacing the pen and paper with human skin, to record family events, such as weddings, births, deaths, etc. Most significant in this respect are some of the customs of Eskimos and African populations, who tattoo on their faces most memorable events experienced by family or tribe.

When examining traditional activities in remote population groups, like in Alaska, Oceania, Mongolia or Madagascar, it is impossible not to see the influence of local religions manifested as specific tattoos. It is this religious component, which was easily adopted by the modern society.

That's how a lot of crosses, crescents, Stars of David, and other much more suggestive symbols, appear everywhere on people's dermis.

The significance of tattoos is based on certain cultural biases, fact which underlines the deep differences between social and anti-social group affiliation. Innocent naïve adolescents offer the image of a restricted group, while criminal street gangs excel in toxicity, when it comes to social order.

In between the two extremes, anyone can find a well-defined, small segment of the society that has no idea why it opted to get tattoos.

WHAT IS A TATTOO?

A tattoo is a form of body mutilation where an epidermal layer is modified by inserting into it, dies, ink or pigments, most of the time permanently. Some modern ways of making them are temporary, yet the most prevalent forms of tattoos are of a permanent nature.

The pigment is injected into the dermis subcutaneous tissue of the skin, sometimes at considerable pain to the bearer.

Many tribal cultures, most notably in Africa, create tattoos by the cutting into the flesh various designs, and rubbing the wound with colored sand, tree sap, or ashes. Sociologists and anthropologists familiar with such customs sustain that this brutal and dangerous method of tattooing did replace the ancestral process of religious sacrifices, widely spread among primitive people. Traditionally, the primitive cultures, all over the world, used tattoos to differentiate the degree of nobility or leadership, in a closed society. The tribe chiefs and their wives were obligated to sport certain types of tattoos to indicate their elite status.

In modern times the tattooing is done by using electric "tattoo machines", which inject ink into the skin with a special needle, or group of needles. The tool for electric tattooing oscillates rapidly, at a rate of 100 to 150 times a second, injecting the desired color pigment.

In many jurisdictions the process of tattooing is strictly regulated in terms of minimum hygiene, and medical standards, age of clients, minimum educations for the tattoo parlor employees, etc.

The corollary health risk factors, both to the client and to operator, are of such a magnitude, that some health authorities spend considerable resources in prevent any epidemics caused by viruses or contaminations acquired during the tattooing process.

The laws in EU countries mandate that a tattoo parlor operator must provide all clients with a printed consent form that describes, in detail, all the risks of complications, providing clear instructions for after care of the wounds.

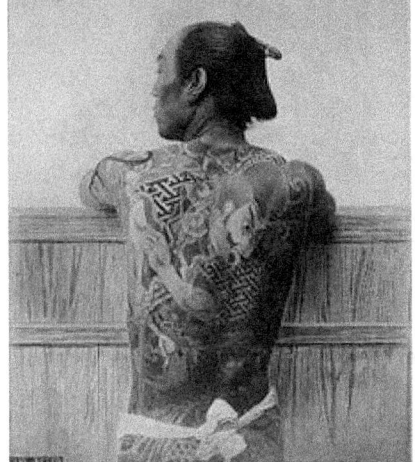

Tattoos on the back of a Japanese mobster

The graphics of tattoo "art" fall in several distinct groups, with clear specifics as to their significance, symbolism, and scope:

Decorative designs, with no symbolic value, only reflect a person's idea of aesthetics, as an element of social differentiation apart from the crowd. Symbolic designs present a definite meaning, relative to wearer's taste and social status. Such graphic schemes indicate, most of the time, spiritual or occupational affiliation, in work, sports, and worship. Extreme designs are meant to frighten certain people, by advertising the fact that the wearer is tough and dangerous. They are a warning for all, that the such a person is capable to inflict pain and suffering to his competitors, or enemies, through gang-assisted beatings, or even by murder.

Originally the custom or the "art" of tattooing was brought to Europe from Polynesia, during the early 18th century, primarily by the sailors of the colonial empires. The tattoos were reserved strictly for men, who "sailed the seven seas". During the 20th century, however, the practice of tattooing was extended, practically, to all levels of the society, including to females, but the stigma of the tattoo culture remained solidly implanted in the minds of most people. The idea that a tattoo was a fashion statement, never took root among educated persons.

Many basic religious tenets consider the human body to be a temple for God, and tattooing it is equivalent to graffiti on Creator's Altar. That's why certain religious denominations, like the Jews, and the Catholics, do prohibit tattooing under any form or meaning. Of course, exceptions abound, especially among those who do not practice the religions they claim to share with others. The Judaism and the Catholicism generally prohibit tattoos based on Biblical commandments spelled out in Leviticus 19. Jews believe that this commandment applies only to Jews.

Most tattoos are permanent, yet it is possible to remove them. One of the Soviet ambassadors to Paris sported some tattoos on his hands and arms, which he acquired while a sailor during World War II and the Kremlin asked him to get rid of all of them. He did that, at a personal cost of over $ 15,000, and a lot of pain.

The level of tattoo acceptance varies from group to group of individuals or organizations. Recently, a chain of fast food restaurants was sued in a federal court for the "discriminating" personnel policies they implemented nationwide.

The management directive was motivated by business needs: "... no applicants will be hired if they have any missing front teeth, or if they have visible tattoos. If you have tattoos, cover them up." **Obviously that was triggered by the sinking public image and, consequently, diminished sales. The plaintiffs lost, as the law suit was tossed out, as baseless and frivolous.**

Such situations will occur more frequently as employers reject the applicants with tattoos.

Obviously, very few customers feel confident being served their food by a youngster with a lot of missing front teeth, and tattoos all over.

Several studies done on tattooed populations and on the society's views on this type of body modifications have revealed some interesting facts: the most popular ages for acquiring tattoos, are between 18 and 29; the least popular ages for getting tattoos are over 50 years of age.

In the past, the Western culture associated tattoos with individuals living on the fringes of the society, however today they are accepted by almost 33% of the population, as a social phenomenon which will only threaten our culture marginally.

The cities with most tattooed people in the USA are Richmond, VA and Houston, TX, where more than 33% of inhabitants have tattoos. Traditionally considered like a form of protest against all sorts of perceived or imagined social inequities, at the beginning of the 21st century, the tattooing began to morph into a form of personal expression, but that goes against the grain of the moral issues that form the basis of our modern civilization.

Some court cases considered tattooing as a form of free speech, thus under Constitutional protection.

Certainly, a tattoo is a very personal form of expression, which may carry with it hidden significance, in terms of social interaction, like in the case of secret organizations, criminal gangs, etc.

Most police departments, all over the world, maintain up to date files with all the tattoos found on convicted criminals, as an easy way to identify and classify them. That helps in determining who the perpetrators, were even in case of death.

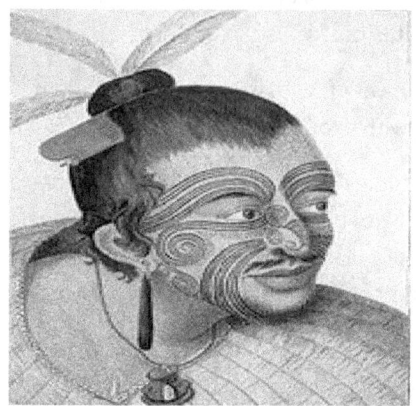

A Maori chief from New Zealand (1935)

The "art" of tattooing was proliferated in almost all countries, in most all social groups, covering most parts of the human anatomy: faces, chests, arms, legs, and even genitals.

Studying the tattoo graphics, one can obtain an accurate image of all human preoccupations, from beliefs, religion, professional characteristics, political views, business orientation, criminal activities, and protests against real or imagined systemic inequities. The consequences of tattooing can be grouped in certain areas of concern, such as:

- Limited options in personal development;

- Limited options in employment;

- Limited opportunities for meaningful social interactions;

- Unlimited health risks augmented by the process of tattooing;

- Unlimited scrutiny from colleagues and customers;

- Unlimited stigma from certain groups of people.

That's why the best advice one can provide to anyone who is contemplating to get tattoos, is to wait a while, until the pressure of the temptation wears off.

If the process of tattooing may be considered by some people, as an ego trip, the consequences of that action can last much longer than the anticipated pleasure of setting oneself apart from the rest of the crowd.

If not evident, this type of action may carry with it many of the elements of a precise reaction, which is rarely positive.

The wearer of tattoos can't be certain of any kind of positive response, more so when it comes to a professional image. For that reason alone, the best advice one can get, is: "If you have tattoos, cover them up!"

The excuse that you were drunk when you stepped into the tattoo parlor is a lame one. You probably didn't think hard enough when you were shown the tattoo artist's images to select from, to get the one that you were convinced it represented the core of your personality, unless you were a gangster, with solid ties to a criminal organization. It would take a long period of time before your "buyer remorse" is extinguished completely, and you realize that you have to live with all the consequences of your tattoo images, for the rest of your life. Such a psychological conundrum offers no solutions to the casual person, who just "invested" into a tattoo, when the "buyer's remorse" sets in.

First, if you consider your tattoo an "investment", you have to realize that the only dividends you'd get would be of a questionable nature. Secondly, your damaged image is only rarely repairable. However, most people realize this fact too late to be able to take corrective measures. Once you jumped in, try to swim.

WHY TATTOOS?

Normally, when one sees a person covered with tattoos several questions come to mind:

"Is that person a jail bird? Are those graphics a form of jail art?"

"Is that person a gang member? Are those tattoos for recognition?"

"Is that person stupid? Are those tattoos proof of lack of judgment?"

The motivation to get tattooed varies, from individual to individual, and in a large measure, falls along the line of a solid "Yes!" answer to all the three questions above. That should not come as a surprise to anyone. People in jails have all the time in the world to compose and execute elaborate tattoos with very primitive tools, since tattooing is against the policies of any US penitentiary. That's why the inmates create their own tattooing devices out of innocent materials they have access to, such as paper clips, staples, ballpoint pens, guitar strings, toothpicks, etc.

The gang members broadcast their affiliation through tattoos, gang colors, clothing accessories, caps and hats. If a gang member fails to display his or her articles of gang identification, the "boss" may impose brutal penalties. That rule will be enforced equally in the jail or outside, on the street. The prevalence of gang colors has declined significantly during the last few years due to crack down by law enforcement and judicial pressure. If a gang member commits a Class "A" Misdemeanor, the highest level of a misdemeanor crime, then that offense will be automatically reclassified as a felony, because the offender is a member of a criminal street gang. Some very vicious gang members have been found to have no tattoos of any kind. Most of the "innocent" tattoos are the result of decisions made on the spur of the moment, under the influence of peers, drugs or alcohol. That would cover most tattoos acquired by soldiers, sailors, or airmen, during their military service. They serve as a reminder of the time spent in one of the military branches, in the Army, Navy, Marine Corps, Air Force or Coast Guard. Recently the Defense Department issued several directives, which do limit the displaying of any tattoo art on all personnel, enlisted or career officers. All those who have visible tattoos have to cover them up, or get rid of them, under the threat of separation, under dishonorable discharge conditions, for disobeying orders.

That proves that a tattoo obtained in the military can turn against some men or women, who had the best intentions. That goes also for those in the civilian life, especially in business. That lack of judgment someone exercised while getting a tattoo, proved to be a negative experience that would extract a relatively high toll for many years to come.

In New York, a freshly graduated MBA person could not secure a decent job anywhere, except as a foreman on a loading dock for a large chain of stores. He had to accept that job, until better prospects would appear. After some two years there he found out from the Human Resources director, that in spite of excellent qualifications, his tattooed arm advertised his lack of judgment, and the company wanted only employees who can prove good judgment and sound decisions.

People get tattoos to advertise their hobbies, religious beliefs, ethnicity, etc., without realizing that the professional success cannot be guaranteed by proclamations on forearm about "I love my dog" next to an image of your Fido.

It is immature or, at least futile, to think otherwise. What do you think of a lady at the Social Security office, working on your case, while displaying a tattoo which says: "Love me or I will kill you"? But this is an extreme example, even though it is real.

If you want to go through the trouble of paying for a tattoo, think twice before you step into that tattoo parlor, and above all, select something tasteful, discreet that would not come to bite you later. Lack of visibility is the best part when it comes to displaying tattoos that are voluntary, since there are some tattoos acquired involuntarily, like in the case of the Jews, marched to gas chambers during the Holocaust. The Nazis tattooed on their forearm the five or six digit registration number.

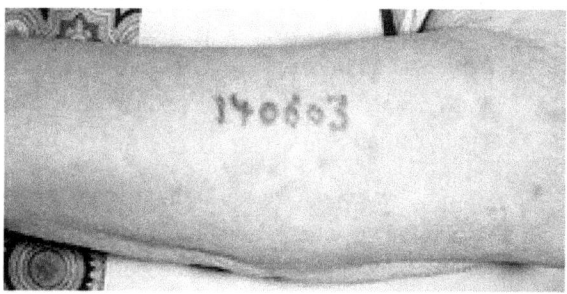

Registration number tattooed on Auschwitz survivor's arm (1942)

For the sake of expediency, the author assumes that most of the tattoos described in this book are voluntary. The people, who went through the pain and the cost of a tattoo parlor artist's work, wanted it done, however, in few cases the tattoos were acquired involuntarily. In that category one has to consider those of the newly inducted crime street gangs, during initiation. The suffering and abject humiliations those youngsters subject themselves to, for the privilege of belonging, are extreme, and the tattoos are proof that they were "men enough to take it".

The graphic styles, their symbolic significance, and the colors used by the gang artists, change constantly. That's why many law enforcement task forces have quite a difficult time identifying and responding to the spread of criminal street gang activities. These gangs continue to incubate and grow constantly new generations of "gangsta" in locales in which no one would suspect this type of high moral contamination.

When there is a certain group of tattoos, and fingerprints are available to identify the members, finding out what they are up to, still requires a lot of special sophisticated police work. In rare cases that is not successful. There always are some attorneys who would jump to defend the worst possible gangsters.

During the Soviet era, criminals sentenced to long terms in Gulag labor camps, tattooed on their chests exceptionally good portraits of Lenin and Stalin, in the mistaken belief that execution squads would not fire into those images.

Some of those criminals had their sentences commuted from death to life in prison, cementing that cruel superstition of "divine protection" from the spirits of Lenin and Stalin.

Some Jews at Auschwitz voluntarily tattooed on their arms swastikas, which spared their lives, and they were not thrown in the incinerators. They were forced instead, to work tending to the death ovens.

Convicts sent to the French tropical penal colonies of Guiana, most notably on the Devil's Island, tattooed on their chests a colorful butterfly, as a memory of the legendary escaped Parisian inmate Henry "Papillon" Charriere. That would maintain alive their hopes of escape. During the 18th and 19th centuries, the British Empire Crown condemned a lot of criminals to "transportation", by banishing them, to the new continent of Australia, with a lifetime interdiction of returning to England. These convicts had a small Union Jack tattooed on the back of their hands, as a warning that such a person was a ward of the King, and was a dangerous criminal. After generations, that became a symbol of pride for the people "transported" to the Australia. Perhaps that is the reason why tattooing has a greater acceptance in Australian than anywhere else.

The practice of tattooing images of the national flag was popular with many other populations, not only among convicts. During World War II, many Japanese prisoners of war displayed the "meat ball", or the Japanese national colors.

There is no consensus among anthropologists and sociologists about the significance of many types of tattoos, yet those designs which incorporate national flags, or nationalistic coat of arms, may represent chauvinism, racism, or hate toward the inhabitants of the neighboring countries. For long time, that psyche survived following the three wars, between Germany and France, between the Soviet Union and the East European countries, between India and China, between Korea and Japan, etc.

During the first years of the 21st century, however, this kind of animosity disappeared, in light of the unionization drive that created the European Union, United Arab Emirates, etc.

Ethnic animosity however, continued to exist in the regions of the former Soviet Union, former Yugoslavia, in Indochina, and in many Muslim counties, even though Islam prohibits tattooing. The graphic subjects of tattoos justified by false national pride or by hate of any other people are rather indicative of the drive to keep all the antagonistic conflicts alive. In this respect, such tattoos represent a "written chronicle" of national viciousness.

JAILBIRDS AND PRISON GANGS

A prison gang is an inmate organization structured like a vast corporation within the prison system, seemingly in perpetuity. All the participating members are "stockholders" in the criminal enterprise. But the membership is restricted along certain ethnic or geographical boundary, requiring a lifetime commitment.

Prison officials and law enforcement professionals refer to prison gangs as the "STGs", or Security Threat Groups, trying to remove any element of gang recognition or publicity, that the gangs crave in order to impose fear among non-member inmates. Such gangs try to force a specific discipline, which frequently results in the murder of non-complying inmates.

There are large, formal, prison gangs, operated based on a "code", which consists in rigid rules, policed by the membership at large. No one is allowed to join, or to transact any business with other prison gangs. Violations are dealt with swiftly and the offenders are routinely murdered.

The prison gangs achieve a social equilibrium based on member loyalty, versus prison guards. The prison yard is minutely divided between various gangs, based on ethnicity, e.g. "for Whites only", "for Blacks only", "for Hispanics only", "for Orientals only", etc. The "stockholders" bind themselves to aid and assist any of their "brothers", but nobody else, through outside connections, mutual aid, loyalty, affection, respect, with a firm standing against the system's rules. Hostility between inmates and prison personnel, fostered through forced restraining of freedom, and lack of access to any heterosexual relationships, creates an environment of hatred and violence, which often erupts in bloody riots.

It seems that the prison administrators thrive on a very high temperature, and a corrupt social environment, with its own political dictates. That's why most inmates can convince prison guards do "small services" for them in procuring contraband. That includes drugs, alcohol, tobacco, money and cell phones.

The prison gangs institute a system of governance with unusual features: well defined property rights inside the prison walls, bartering with the outside world, exchanges of "favors", such as "investments", and many other functions normally reserved for bona-fide corporate entities.

As an example, the prison gang known as the Mexican Mafia yields enough power to control the drug dealers on the street. Of course, the street dealers all benefit from that, and gladly pay the jail gang-imposed protection tax.

The prison gangs provide some specific services, in and out of the jail. They protect their dealers while incarcerated, or while on the street, and settle any disputes.

The prison gangs hold some sort of monopoly on violence, both inside and outside the jails. This way they can easily extort considerable sums of money from outside gangs, while some of their members are incarcerated, effectively using such street gang members as hostages. The prison gang diplomacy includes open actions to encourage certain street gangs to steal from, and to start wars with other non-taxpaying street gangs, most notably rival gangs.

The animosity between White and Black gangs, or between Hispanic and Oriental gangs, often degenerates into full scale prison riots, which often require the intervention of the law enforcement formations, like State Police, or the National Guard units.

The gang members use coded communications with their partners who are on the street, and the prison officials have a hard time deciphering their letters or phone calls.

Generally, most all the prison gangs are ripe for picking as recruitment cadres, for Islamic "missionaries", most commonly among Black inmates. Many imams will commit minor offenses, to be sentenced to short jail terms, just to have the opportunity to recruit "new blood".

The ability of some prison gang members to do a certain type of "public relations" work, inside the jail walls, is amazing. They work quite well to enlarge their basis of operations, outside, on the street, and constantly seek to gain new adherents, mostly along the ethnic lines established by the "leadership".

The constant struggle between certain prison gangs often is relaxed, in order to achieve a questionable peace, time in which the violence between archrivals is discouraged. That happens often during Christian holidays or during the Muslim Ramadan.

The prison officials work feverishly, to find out what exactly happens since they are used to encounter calm weather before a violent stormy period hits.

It is the conclusion of the specialists who study prison gangs that it is virtually impossible to eliminate gang activities in the jail, no matter what kind of measures are employed. Dangerous inmates dispersed through the entire country, in maximum security prisons, will continue to "work" their schemes in spite of intelligence data collected on them. Prison gangs develop rapidly outside connections which are richly advertised through specific tattoos, even if all the correctional institutions prohibit tattooing.

WHITE PRISON GANGS

The Aryan Brotherhood was started in early 1960s in the California prison system, and only accepts as members, white American inmates. Estimated to number about 2,000 members, is the smallest prison gang, yet most powerful in terms of "assets" controlled in and out of prison. It cultivates successfully a reputation of ruthlessness and violence.

It has an emblem, "the brand", of a white shield with a green shamrock and the number "666", next the letters "AB" ("Aryan Brotherhood"). Since 2001 this gang has been targeted heavily by state and federal authorities, and most of its members have been dispersed all over the country, in maximum security units.

Surprisingly enough, the authorities in Utah discovered stashes of drugs and cash valued at over $ 100,000, in spite of frequent and minute searches. The inmates involved were separated and sent to different prisons. It is suspected that such actions from the part of the gang members could not have been carried out without the support and knowledge of some prison guards.

The Nazi Low Riders are a relatively new prison gang, formed after most of the leaders of the Aryan Brotherhood have been sent to the Pelican Bay or Rikers Island prisons. This gang accepts only White members, including Italian and Hispanic ones, who are light-skinned, able to pass as Caucasians. Typically this small prison gang does not get involved with drugs. They prefer to deal in stolen vehicles and auto parts, facts for which they all receive smaller sentences. They control several car dealerships, in California, Nevada, and in Arizona, posing in good corporate citizens. Their modus operandi involves "saving" auto dealerships in financial trouble. In exchange for their "loans", they are allowed to "skim" up to 10% of the gross income. Usually such dealerships end up bankrupt.

The European Kindred is a prison gang founded in Oregon in 1970, and it is affiliated with the Aryan Brotherhood and with the Ku Klux Klan. This organization gets its money through the extortion of other inmates, or their families. This gang is known for torture and murder of inmates, who do not join them.

The Brotherhood of Aryan Alliance, also known as the 211's, and the 13K, or the "Killers of MS 13" is a small prison gang formed and operating since 2001, in the plain state penitentiaries, in Texas, Oklahoma, Kansas, Arkansas and Iowa. No one knows exactly how many members are there, or how they derive their income in order to survive financially, as a gang.

The Aryan Circle prison gang was formed in the East Coast jails, and it is a small fringe offshoot of the original Aryan Brotherhood, numbering less than 500 members, and it is active both in and out of the prison walls. It is concerned with domination over minorities, being deeply involved in the drug trade. This gang is quite vicious, in eliminating real and imaginary enemies.

The Dead Man Incorporated, or the DMI, was founded in late 1990 in the Maryland prison system, with followers all over the US. It boasts about of a large membership of over 1,000 followers. It conducts a brisk business in loansharking to other gangs peddling drugs.

The Aryan Brotherhood of Texas, or the ABT, does not have direct ties with the original Aryan Brotherhood, and it operates as a criminal enterprise. Founded in 1980s, it has a membership list of approximately 3,000 people, all recruited from the white population of Texas inmates. It works "contracts of elimination" for anyone who could pay $ 10,000 to have someone killed. The drug trade is only a small part of its business, next to illegal gambling, and prostitution. They will finance the purchase of gambling machines for filling stations and truck stops, for exorbitant rates. These gambling machines being illegal in Texas, often end up confiscated and destroyed by the authorities, leaving their owners "in hock" to the financing gangs for long periods of time. Failure to pay back the loans results in harsh punishment, including murder. More recently, it has been found that some of the "financing" gangs obtain substantial life insurance policies on their victims, just before they are killed by unknown persons. But, on the other hand, several other criminal gangs get their income from insurance fraud, a situation in which most innocent people have to foot the bills. They are adept at "staging" automobile crashes, in which they collect impressive amounts of money from insurance companies. It is suspected that certain corrupt policemen support such acts.

These criminal gangs rarely use the court systems, and when they do, they find attorneys that provide them legal services. In the state of Florida, such a gang racked more than 5 million dollars in less than three years. During the trial it resulted that several of the local policemen were paid "kickbacks" for every accident report filed for the gang members. In one certain case, a gang member backed his vehicle into the car of a federal judge, and, a policeman wrote an accident report without knowing exactly who the victim was. The accident report stated that the victim failed to control his vehicle and ran into the other person's vehicle. A surveillance video camera, from the front of the courthouse revealed a different picture. After FBI investigations, it was discovered immediately that the same five or so gang members collected enormous sums of money from several insurance companies, for such staged accidents.

BLACK PRISON GANGS

The Bloods, also known as the "RBG", or the Ruthless Blood Gang, was originally a criminal street gang, but after multiple arrests it was relegated to the status of a black prison gang. Initially this all-Black gang was formed to protect members from the rival Crips. It engaged in all sorts of illegal activities, from drug smuggling, to contract killing. In early 2000s it was absorbed by the United Blood Nation gang with a wide representation inside and outside the jails from the western USA.

The Black Guerilla Family is a prison gang founded in 1966, at San Quentin State Prison, in California, initially meant as a political civil rights movement, by the late Black Panther member George L. Jackson (1941 – 1971). It is estimated that today this gang has a membership of some 1,500 people. Initially, this gang was conceived to raise its money through legitimate business activities however, after the death of its founder the drug trade appeared much more appealing.

The Crips are also a Black gang which originally operated in the Los Angeles area, often getting into bloody conflicts with the Bloods.
Estimated to number over 3,000 members, its members move constantly in and out of jails, fact for which they are considered a strictly prison gang. Their sphere of activity encompasses drugs, human trafficking, bank robberies, prostitution, loansharking and contract killing. They are on an open path of war with the local police, since early beginnings in 1969.

The United Blood Nation was a Black prison gang on the East Coast, in state jails. In early 2000s, following infiltration by special state and federal agents, this criminal organization was just about completely obliterated. However, this gang was regenerated by the

Bloods, when they joined the Crips in the Western US. They are estimated to number around 2,000 members.

The Folk Nation or the People's Nation is a prison gang operating in the Midwest and South, currently allied with other criminal street gangs, most notably with the Bloods. They deal in narcotics, prostitution, contract killing, and loansharking.

The D.C. Blacks is a loosely-knit criminal organization founded in the Washington D.C. prison system, by Islamic missionaries, who recruited them and trained them in the Jihad ideology. They are sworn enemies of the Aryan Brotherhood, Mexican Mafia, and of the Jewish gang, the Yiddish Black Hand. The members of this gang would do everything possible to destroy the western society, because of its corruption by alcohol, narcotics and politics. It is often suspected that upon release from prison many members of this gang are relocated to Muslim countries, where they are trained in Arabic and Islamic religious concepts.

The Islam discourages tattooing, yet the former gang members are allowed to keep them under a special religious "Fatwa", (religious dispensation), issued by the ISIS Islamic Council. The relations between various Black gangs and Muslims are unpredictable: some "season" they all cooperate to import drugs from Mexico, while other times they kill each other in fierce battles for turf, resulting in numerous deaths.

They all carry sophisticated weapons, from UZIs to NK-47 and all are capable to stage bloody confrontations with the local police or with sheriff departments.

Some spectacular bank robberies were perpetrated by them, as were some spectacular mass shootings of innocent civilians.

HISPANIC PRISON GANGS

MS-13, or Mara Salvatrucha, simply the MS or the Mara, is an international criminal organization started in, in Costa Rica, spread throughout the entire western hemisphere.

Extremely vicious, this gang kills indiscriminately anyone in their way, in order to terrorize people into submission to their crime schemes. There is no field of criminal activity in which MS-13 is not represented, from drugs to identification theft, and bank fraud. It is estimated that MS-13 has a membership in excess to 50,000 people, with half of them active in Los Angeles and San Francisco areas. As a criminal street gang, its members are affiliated for life, under the penalty of death in case of desertion. It is estimated that the MS-13 collects over $ 10,000,000 monthly, which facilitates bribing officials in several countries.

The US law enforcement organs are in a constant state of war with MS-13, but, at this time, it is difficult to ascertain who wins and who loses.

La Eme Gang, or the Mexican Mafia, is named after the 13th letter of the Latin alphabet, "M", based on the superstition that Jesus had 12 Apostles, for a total group of 13 followers, thus they may benefit from good luck. This gang is composed mostly of Hispanics, although there are some White members. Many times the Mexican Mafia is allied with the White Brotherhood in order to share in the profits made in the narcotics trade, gun-running, prostitution, and "hits" on a contract basis. With a territory encompassing most of the southern states, from Florida to California, this gang rakes impressive profits from activities managed from inside the prisons. They excel in drug distribution, in selection of bank robbery targets, fencing stolen goods, trailer hijacking, protection rackets, etc.

Latin Kings Gang or the "Reyes Del Norte", is a California-based street criminal organization, which accepts only Hispanic members. In order to join, a candidate has to murder one person selected by the boss, the El Rey. The membership is for life and any attempt to leave the brotherhood is punished by death. This criminal gang works extremely closely with the Mexican drug smugglers, raking in substantial profits in the California. During the last decade, this gang got into fierce battles with the Creeps and the Bloods over the turf in which all of them deal in human trafficking, prostitution, and illegal arms. It is estimated that the Latin Kings have a total membership of less than 3,000 men and women, and are well represented outside California in larger cities like New York, Miami, Chicago, Houston, and Philadelphia. They accept women as second-class members subject to the same rules as the men. Their code of silence is enforced to extremes, fact which explains the large number of murders among their own gang members.

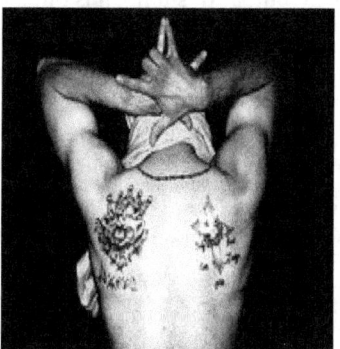

Latin Kings member showing coat of arms and cross tattoos (1999).

The Nuestra Familia Gang, ("Our Family"), was first established in the California's Soledad prison in early 1960s, and represents some criminals originating in Mexico, or in the mostly rural areas of the southern California. Many of them cannot speak English.

Their main sources of income are derived from the importation of narcotics from Mexico. Members of this gang have the lowest life expectancy of all prison gangs, at around 19 years of age.

The Texas Syndicate is a prison gang that recruits its member from the ranks of illegal Mexican aliens spending time in Texas jails. . The main source of income is originated by extortion, most of the time from the families of those inmates that they would court for membership. No Whites or Blacks are ever allowed to live or work in their "barrios". ("Turf")

The Netas Gang is primarily a Puerto Rico prison gang, with very little representation in US, except for New York, Miami, and Philadelphia jails. This criminal organization numbers less than 500 people and prefers to deal in arms and stolen automobiles.

The Sepulcro Gang ("Tomb") is a prison gang originated in Mexico and spread through incarcerated illegal aliens in US. Their "brand" tattoo is a coffin, signifying certain death if crossed. They worship the Santa Muerte, ("The Saint Death"), as their protector. They number less than 1,000 men, but commit, almost 100% of the drug war murders, on both sides of the Rio Grande, which forms the border with Mexico. The great majority of this gang's members are less than 20 years old. Their main sources of income consist in the drug trade profits, protection rackets, prostitution, and thefts of merchandise from railroad cars. This gang is extremely elusive, according to American law enforcement organs.

Cooperation among Hispanic gangs is quite rare, however, during the last few years, after 2015, the law enforcement organs detected a strong drive for uniting several prison gangs.

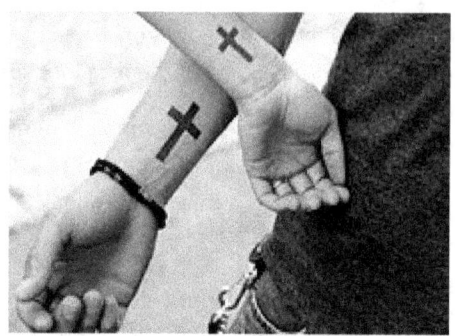

Crosses tattooed on the arms of a "Christian" gang member (1998)

The Hispanic gangs, in Mexico and in Honduras, draw inspiration in their tattoo graphics from the rich folklore of the Aztec culture. That includes in large part, mythology and astrology. Consequently a lot of tattoos are based on various standards rooted in ancient beliefs. That translates in the "signs", which indicate a gang member's status and function, along the "business" lines practiced.

These "signs" are indicative of a marriage between ancient folklore and the modern gang life. They may be executed in black, blue or red ink, and serve as a positive identification of gang members. These "signs" are quite suggestive:

Alligator, a determined, loyal member of the "community;

Wind, a man of mobility, who adapts rapidly to changing conditions;

House, a rock-solid temper, who does not allows for ambiguity;

Lizard, a hiding artist, elusive and adept at changing colors;

Serpent, a leading member of the gang;

Death, an intrinsic part of life which always follows the birth;

Deer, an inhabitant of rural areas that can guide to "meat";

Rabbit, resilient escape artist;

Water, a person of fluidity who knows the secrets of gang life;

Dog, a dependable ally that can warn of coming danger;

Monkey, an untrustworthy member of the gang fraternity;

Grass, person in charge with processing marijuana for sale;

Reed, boss man;

Ocelot, effective hunter of "enemies of the gang";

Eagle, person in charge with overseeing gang discipline;

Vulture, person charged with disposing of dead bodies;

Earthquake, sworn to total destruction;

Knife, enforcer of gang discipline;

Rain, favorite member, in line for leadership in the gang;

Flower, new person, usually a female, just accepted in the gang.

    Somehow, certain elements of ancient Aztec mythology and astrology permeated throughout the ages, in spite of fierce battles with the Catholic establishments of Mexico or Honduras, and were adopted by the underground movement of criminal gangs. Soon the imagery and the themes of the Aztecs, materialized into colorful tattoos, which found their way into many penal institutions, including those in the USA.

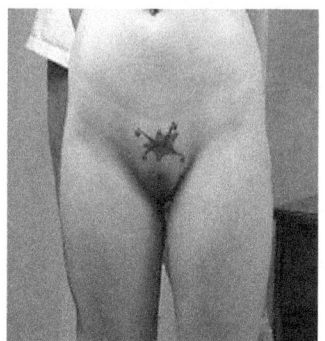

Genital tattoos on a female member of the Latin Kings.

This type of tattoo indicates that this female had intercourse with all gang members, and that she became one of the most trusted confidants of the "boss". Such women are well versed in criminal activities, and are capable of horrible acts, from mutilation, to murder through torture, and beheading.

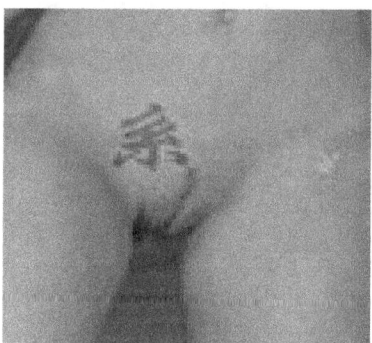

Genital tattoo on a woman considered property of the Triad gang.

The Chinese caption, taken from a Kung Fu, (Confucius), classic text, states boldly that: "By pleasing others, you get closer to

Heaven". Such female gang members are a vital part of the Chinese crime culture and are expected to finish successfully any of the tasks assigned by the gang boss. Such tasks may consist in drug smuggling, bank fraud, or in contract killings.

The law enforcement organs on mainland China, or in Taiwan, are often at a point that they hardly can believe the savagery with which such women transact the gang business. Posing in innocent, naïve ladies of the night, they are easily able to penetrate companies and institutions, as insiders for the benefit of the Triad. In a well-known case in Hong Kong, such a female gang member was able to poison all the employees on a certain floor of a large bank, after which she absconded with impressive sums of money. Even though videotaped by the security cameras, the police had a difficult time identifying the female perpetrator, because she used elaborate disguises, such as wigs, and unobtrusive clothing. By studying such cases, one may be inclined to conclude that there is no difference between various types of crime. That spectrum starts with city prostitution and spans the whole field of illegal activities. That justifies fully the Chinese swift administration of death penalty in all similar cases.

The Chinese government is sincerely interested in stamping out organized crime, in order to foster an atmosphere conducive to foreign investments and healthy business. The Mao regime was able to eliminate the Triad organizations by executing their members. The few survivors selected to live in exile, in India, Vietnam, Thailand, Taiwan, or in Latin America. The few remaining old members are currently working to reestablish a much more modern Triad criminal gang, using modern technology in order to penetrate the banking systems. So far, according to various police reports, their presence is apparent in significant numbers.

RUSSIAN CRIMINAL GANGS

The Russian prison gangs, called "Vory" in Russian, is an experienced organization established during the Gulag era, and continued to be active long after release from the notorious labor camps. Many members emigrated to the West, and reached USA and Canada, where they engaged in lucrative crime endeavors. The Russian community in USA denies the existence of any Russian criminal gangs here, claiming that they shall be called "Jewish criminal gangs from Russia".

The Russian criminal gang enforce a strict code of "ethics" as "thieves in law". According to that code, no one is allowed to get tattoos without the express approval of the "Glova", the head man.

Under this code of the V*ory*, a thief must:

- Never show his emotions;
- Forsake his relatives: father, mother, brothers, sisters, etc.;
- Not have any family of his own: no marriage, no children; this does not, however, preclude him from having an unlimited number of concubines. During a large gathering of thieves-in-law, during the late 1980s, this rule was removed.
- Never, under any circumstances, have a legitimate job or significant property (e.g. a house), no matter how much difficulty this can bring; live only on money obtained through gambling or theft, and rely on lower-level criminal connections for food or accommodations. The word 'theft' as used here describes any criminal activity considered 'legitimate' by the Vory. the 'head thief-in-law' has a leadership position, so direct participation in arms smuggling or drug trafficking is totally incompatible with such a high status, since those activities are a form of commerce. However receiving tribute from smugglers and drug-dealers, or robbing and extorting them, is a legitimate activity for a 'thief-in-law' (Traditional thieves still respect this rule but the modern Vory tends to be involved only in the more

lucrative positions, but this rule now, is relatively ignored in the regions outside Siberian prison camps.)
- Help other thieves: both by moral and material support, by utilizing your connections in the commune of thieves;
- Rule and arbitrate the criminal world and protect basic needs of criminals and prisoners, according to the extents and priorities set by the thieves' commune (typically in a given prison/prison cell, or region, even outside, when not imprisoned);
- Keep secret all the information about the whereabouts of your comrades (e.g. dens, districts, hideouts, safe apartments, etc.).
- In unavoidable situations (if a thief is under investigation or is arrested) take the blame for someone else's crime; this buys the other person time to escape and remain free. Demand an inquiry and judgment by a council of thieves to resolve disputes in the event of a conflict between oneself and other thieves;
- If necessary, participate in such inquiries, if called upon;
- Punish any offending thief as decided by the judgment of the thieves' council. Do not resist carrying out the decision of punishment for the offending thief who is found guilty;
- Have a good command of the thieves' slang (called "Fenya"), a distinct language spoken by hardcore criminals in Russia, and understood only by few outsiders. Never gamble without being able to cover your losses.
- Teach the criminal way of life to youth with good potential;
- Have, if possible, informants from the rank and file of thieves. Do not to lose your reasoning abilities when drunk.
- Have nothing to do with the authorities (particularly with the CLU, Correctional Labor Authority), do not participate in public activities, nor join any community organizations. (This rule came from the Soviet era and rarely applies now)
- Not serve in the military or accept any weapons from the government or prison authority (police batons). (Again this rule rarely applies today, in fact, the Vory men control the black market, which is full of discharged Soviet military weapons)
- Make good on promises given to other thieves.
- Never deny your Vory status directly. To the questions like 'Are you a Vory?' or "Why are you a lifer?", a Vory should always answer: "Yes, I am a Vory!", or, "Because I killed someone who asked too many questions", even if asked by police and the

encounter is videotaped. The latter question phrase is ritual and video footage containing the answer is sometimes used by the Russian authorities to justify Vory arrests for the media (not very common, though).

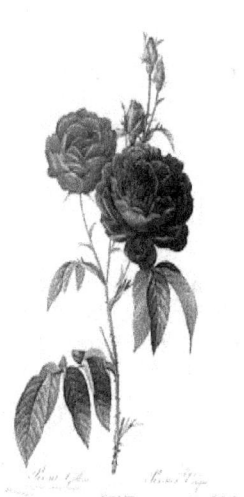 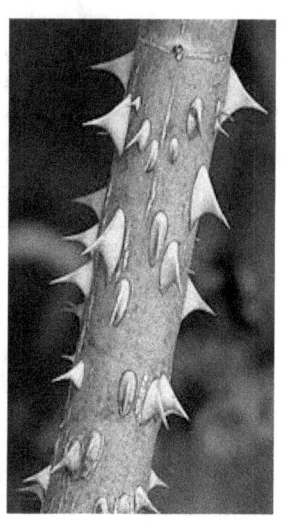

               1935   1939

Details of tattoo templates used by Russian inmates.

A rose symbolized the full opposition to the communism during the Soviet era, and a total disregard for the behavioral rules of the modern society of today's Russia.

Allegations of close cooperation between Vory and the Muslim separatists or "jihad" in Russia are, most likely, false. The Russian gangsters are primarily xenophobic and do not tolerate to have any members of foreign extraction. They use brutal fascist methods to prevent "pollution" with foreigners.

ORIENTAL CRIMINAL GANGS

The Japanese, Chinese, Korean and the Vietnamese gangs, operating in and out of US prisons, are some inpenetrable criminal entities, which seem inscrutable to most law enforcement agencies. That is due primarily to language barriers, and to their cultural idiosyncrasies.

They include Yakuza and Gokudo, as the most representative member of the Japanese Mafia. The Chinese crime syndicate known as the Triad, is active in Shanghai, Hong Kong and Taipei. The South Korean criminal gangs are relatively independent, while some of the crime activities seem to be organized by the North Korean authorities similar in work style to a "fifth column", engaged in government-sponsored "hits". The Vietnamese gang members, while not in jail, prefer to "work" in ports of entry for all sorts of goods, including arms and drugs. The author was unable to locate verifiable source regarding any data about some of these oriental gangs, but their presence is well known.

The telling signs of the oriental criminal gangs, especially in the restrictive Chinatowns, or in the areas with large numbers of people transplanted from Asiatic countries, can only be verified after the arrest, and sentencing of perpetrators, for serious felonies. The preferred areas of activity are around ports and fishing fleets, where, at times, they engage local people in armed conflicts. Such Oriental gang members try to muscle in on local labor unions and on fishing fleet operators. Heists of trailer loaded with high-value merchandise, bank robberies in small towns, and unexplained homicides, all bear the unquestionable mark of the oriental gang activities. They are vicious, preferring to torture their victims before killing them. Such gangs enforce a strict code of silence when it comes to interaction with outsiders or with the law agencies.

That gives them an edge above their rivals.

One of their main rules, enforced to limits, is the prohibition of killing police officers, in order to avoid attracting attention.

The gangs from Taiwan set up "hacking training centers" where they try to form reliable computer hackers, ready to attack the most sophisticated IT centers, in order to steal vital information. It is suspected that, most spectacular security breaches in bank customer lists come from penetrated proprietary data bases. In 2016 some 50 million accounts have been hijacked and auctioned off on sections of the dark Web. These computer hackers are flexible, sophisticated, and ruthless. The bulk of the Oriental gang members rarely get sentenced to prison terms, since they can afford to retain the services of the best law firms.

In 2014, Wang Liu, a Hong Kong resident, was arrested in England for the offense of trafficking in information stolen from data bases belonging to the largest international corporations. After two years, he was let go free, because of "lack of credible evidence".

In order to complete the list of prison gangs operating in and out of the jails of the EU, Russia, and Eastern Europe, one has to consider the Irish Mafia, Russian Mafia, Jewish Mafia, Italian Mafia, Georgian Mafia, and the Romanian Mafia, all organized in a loose brotherhood of drug purveyors, extortionists, arsonists, human traffickers, weapons smugglers, contract killers, and thieves of data. Local police units and the Interpol try to compile a realistic picture of the structure and extent of the spread of organized crime activities worldwide, so far with limited success.

Chinese Triad Societies are some of the oldest criminal organizations in the world, with uninterrupted activities since 1800s.

A Triad is one of many branches of a Chinese transcontinental organized crime syndicate, active in Hong Kong, Macau, Taiwan, and also in countries with significant Chinese populations, such as the USA, Canada, UK, Vietnam, Korea, Japan, Singapore, Philippines,

Indonesia, Malaysia, Thailand, Belgium, Netherlands, France, Spain, South Africa, and Australia. The starting point for understanding Chinese triads is to make a clear distinction between the Taiwan Triad and mainland Chinese criminal organizations. In the ancient Chinese traditions, a Triad was only one of the three major secret societies known as Wang, Wu and Wuidao. It created branches in Macau, Hong Kong, Taiwan and Chinese communities overseas. After the establishment of the People's Republic of China, all secret societies were completely destroyed in mainland China, through a series of campaigns organized by Chairman Mao. Although post-Mao China has witnessed the resurgence of organized crime groups, they are no longer classical triad societies; the proper term for these criminal organizations is "mainland Chinese criminal organizations", which consist of two major types of organizations: the dark forces (loosely organized groups) and the black societies (more mature criminal organizations). Two features that distinguish a black society from a dark force are (1) the ability of achieving illegal control over local markets, and (2) the obtainment of police protection. In short, Hong Kong triad refers to traditional criminal organizations operating in or originating from Hong Kong, Macau, Taiwan and in Southeast Asian countries, while organized crime groups in mainland China are better called "mainland Chinese criminal gangs". They deal primarily with the import-export of narcotics, human trafficking, loansharking, illegal gambling, and prostitution.

    What is remarkable about the Chinese Triads is the fact that they were able to survive the Mao regime, by joining the Chinese Communist Party, with many gang members reaching high positions in the Chinese government. Triads currently engage in a variety of crimes from fraud, extortion, and money laundering, to trafficking and prostitution. They also are involved in smuggling and in the counterfeiting of products, such as music CDs, video, software, as well as more tangible goods, like apparel, watches, and currency ney.

For recognition, the Chinese Triads and the Japanese Yakuza members, amputate their small finger on the left hand.

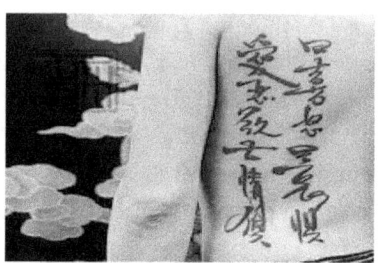

Cursive calligraphy of a Chinese gang tattoo, stating in Mandarin: "The honor of the oat keeper is like a shining star." (1970)

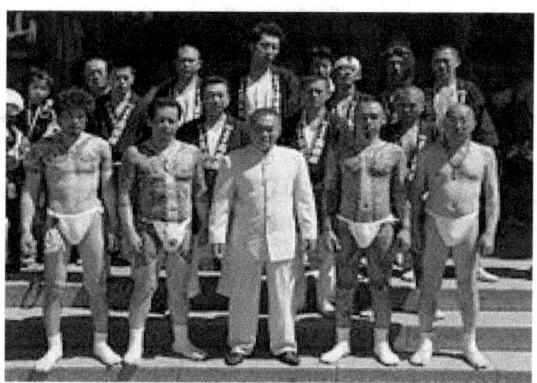

Japanese Yakuza gang members showing off tattoos. (1988)

According to the latest data regarding gang activities in the US, the current administration is poised to help all the law enforcement agencies to stamp out criminal gangs. During the first half of 2018 over 10,000 gang members from California and New York were arrested and or deported.

Some of the prominent oriental gangs, formed in the US after the end of the Vietnam war consisted in Vietnamese immigrants, belonging to certain clans, such as the Sichuan Clan, Yunnan Clan, and Guangxi families. They proudly called themselves "Hmong" and formed a loosely-knit group of people operating on the fringes of the American society. They were supported by the US government's largess in the name of pluralism, and as such, they never integrated into the USA modern society. They still practice the slavery and forcefully coerce minor into prostitution.

Inability to speak English, after more than 30 years here, has reduced their field of criminal activities to the immigrant Southwestern Asia populations, primarily from Laos and Vietnam. They prohibit the use of drugs in their "family", but are glad to sell them to their established clientele. They did not like to establish themselves in large cities, preferring to live in isolated rural areas, where the law enforcement organs are not sophisticated enough to annihilate Asiatic gang activities or to penetrate them.

During the 1980s these Asiatic gangs, especially those of Vietnamese origin started "wars" with the local fishermen in many areas on the southern Gulf Coast.

The struggle for turf in lucrative Gulf fishing areas soon degenerated in armed conflicts which ended in deaths on both sides. The Vietnamese "families" attempted to take over the oyster banks, by ignoring local rules and regulations and, finally destroying the habitat, so that no one could make a living fishing there. Some specialists sustain that transplanting foreign populations in the USA, is equivalent to the process of introduction of invasive species in the local ecosystem which results in irreversible biological damages.

Very few of the transplanted criminal societies into the USA would ever assimilate.

Typical in this sense is the fact that most Oriental gangs keep one of their prominent members as translators and representatives when dealing with the local officials. They are truly advocates for the gangs, when they apply for welfare. Subsequently many of the gang members benefit of the largess of the American taxpayer, in using rent subsidies, food stamps, scholarships for their children, and any of the money available to fight poverty.

America is the only country in the world, where gang members drive brand new cars and trucks, to pick up their welfare checks, while "scoring" impressive illegal income.

How can our state and federal governments, and the local law enforcement agencies tolerate such a paradox? Simply by the inability to create any kind of realistic image of the secretive Oriental gangs. They have far too few employees fluent in the respective languages, while the imported cultures prevent meaningful interaction through a rigid silence code.

Only the members of the second or third generation of immigrant criminal gang families would leave for larger cities, like Yew York, Chicago, Los Angeles or Houston, the rest of them, the aging gangsters, continue to remain in the local area where they settled first. That reduces rather considerably their "opportunities" for additional victims, thus income.

The reduction in crime is due primarily to attrition.

HIDDEN MEANING OF TATTOOS

Most gang members, whether in detention or free, display tattoos all over their bodies, for member identification, or as substitute for the Curriculum Vitae of their career in the crime industry.

The following list of tattoo graphics tries to group them in an ascending succession, from simple to complex:

Aztec mythology figures: **Texas Syndicate form of recognition;**

One dot on hand: **I escaped once;**

Two dots on hand: **I attempted to escape twice;**

Three dots on hand: **I will succeed on my third escape attempt;**

Dots on hands: **signify the number of years spent in jail;**

One teardrop **under the right eye: killed one policeman;**

Two teardrops **under the right eye: killed more than one policeman;**

One teardrop **under the left eye: killed one person**   Two Teardrops **under the left eye: lost a loved gang "brother";**

Barbed wire on arms: **sentenced to minor jail term for a felony;**

Barbed wire on legs: **unjustly sentenced to a short jail term;**

Barbed wire on forehead: **life sentence without parole;**

Swastika on forehead: **revenge on inferior races;**

Swastika on arms: **warrior against inferior races;**

Heart with dagger: **will kill spouse or girlfriend, if not loyal;**

Cross: **will not obey anyone except God;**

Cross on forehead: **inmate on Death Row;**

Dollar sign on the inside of palm: **loan shark;**

Duck on chest: **survived murder attempt;**

Fish on the back, **signifies survival at any cost;**

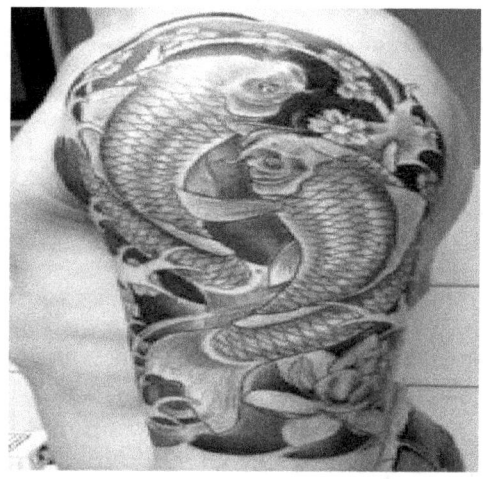

Bun Hui tattoo of Koi fish, signifies a high ranking Triad member of the Hong Kong gang

Star on chest: **leader of the gang;**

Star on knee: **will not kneel in front of no one;**

Star on genitals: **favorite sex partner for the gang boss;**

Flower on chest: **fully accepted "sister";**

Tombstone on back: **time lost due to the corrupt justice;**

CC on Russian gang members: **German SS symbol;**

Cactus on left arm: **will cooperate with the law against Black gangs;**

Cactus on right arm: **will cooperate with the law against White gangs;**

Diamond on forehead: **will issue contract on prison guard(s);**

Two diamonds on forehead: **prison guard killed under contract;**

Three diamonds on forehead: **money paid for contract to kill;**

Elephant on chest: **will always remember those who deserve to die;**

Frog on hand: **will survive hail or high water;**

Goose on arm: **punished with solitary confinement;**

Horse or mule on arms: **drug courier for the gang;**

"Incluido": **("Included", in Spanish") outstanding member;**

Jackrabbit on back: **kicked out of a rival gang;**

"Kilo" on shoulder; **extremely successful cocaine dealer;**

Longhorn on chest: **affiliation with the Texas Syndicate;**

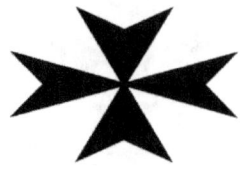

Malta Cross

Malta Cross on chest: **Christian gang soldier;**

Malta Cross on arms: **former gang boss;**

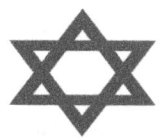

Mogen David

Mogen David on chest: **("David's Star") Jewish gang soldier;**

Menorah on chest: **Faith and law soldier;**

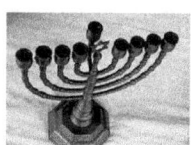

Menorah

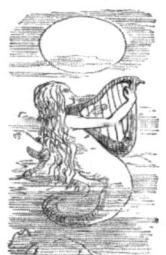

Mermaid

Mermaid on back: **crossed Rio Bravo several times, with drugs;**

Ninety nine (99) on hand: **chief settler of disputes in jail, or on the street;**

Oyster on arms: **claim for "tax" on Gulf oyster banks fished by Vietnamese;**

Quill on the arm: **collector of debts for fellow members;**

Peacock on the back: **pimp;**

Rooster or ram on arms: **pimp;**

Snake on arms or legs: **enforcer of gang rules;**

Tiger on shoulder: **Triad gang boss;**

"Unido": **("United" in Spanish), merged gang member;**

Vampire bat: **Bled someone to death;**

"Pancho" Villa on chest: **Mexican Mafia boss;**

Whip on arms or legs: **Mexican Mafia enforcer;**

"Xavier" on forearm: **under the protection of St. Francis;**

"Z" on hands: **member of the Mexican Zetas gang;**

Aside from the above tattoos, there are scores of graphic representations of gang affiliation, rank, and function, from soldier to boss, and judge, in essence going parallel to the civil structure of today's society. A number of interesting symbols and depiction of Aztec mythological figures find their way in the interlope world, primarily among the Hispanic gang members. However, the gangs populating Central America and Mexico will follow loosely the model of the Aztec society, as recorded over the last centuries, by the Spanish priests, or the Conquistadors.

The variety of graphic details in gang membership, tries to legitimize the task of penetrating the modern society, for obtaining illicit income, and to seed fear in those who violate the gang "codes". Popular in this respect is a pair of red tattoos on both sides of the mouth, of a dagger and a pair of lips. That is a direct reminder, to the membership, that breaking the silence code, (lips), will most likely end up in the offender's death, (dagger).

Some police department collected impressive collections of photographs depicting the naked bodies of gang members covered in tattoos.

Intelligence departments classify and document successfully most of those tattoos, as to their origination, style, and meaning.

Since the tattoos are a social phenomenon here to stay, it is advised that all the persons in charge of hiring new employees to have a basic knowledge of the type and significance of the tattoo graphics observed. It is much better to avoid hiring a jailbird or a gang member, than to handle the aftermath of the damages created in a commercial organization.

The inherent damages of hiring questionable people range from theft, to arson, murder, or to other types of grave crimes.

Most large companies offer specific training to Human Resources employees in order to facilitate valid screening methods that would shield them from liability, as far as any of the possible charges of discrimination may be concerned. It has been well documented, through court actions, that administering complex pre-employment tests to any candidates for employment, does not violate their civil rights, even if some attorney claim that such tests place minorities at a disadvantage. That is true in many situations in which Blacks, Hispanics and immigrants have a poor command of the English language or can't read or write properly.

The argument that hiring a poorly educated employee causes serious problems is a valid one, and that goes hand in hand with the visible tattoos. Such people will not integrate into the company culture, and would not be sincere, no matter what position they occupy. That is a generalization which does not account for possible exceptions. That's why a person with authority in the chain of command of any economic enterprise, or in any institution, has to assert the meaning of the graphics tattooed on the exposed parts of someone's body. That can save a lot of heart aches to all.

It is a known fact that criminal minds are constantly on a look out for opportunities to "score", under the cover of the notion of fulltime employment. That's why the security considerations are so vital to safeguard the income stream.

The tattoos may tell a story about the wearer which is not quite rosy, which could stab at the very heart of any economic operation, however, the person in charge has to become familiar with all such details.

No matter how vigilant one is, when it comes to collective assets or income, attacks will occur under the best safeguards. Usually when the damages are done, it is too late to undo what could have been easily prevented, simply by properly interpreting the tattoos a new employee may display.

There are no such things as insignificant details when dealing with people with a recent criminal past, be it from the part of a street gang member, or a recently released jailbird. Statistically the ratio of honest people to criminals is better than 100 to 1, yet when you happen to come across that one statistical element, the mishap is always due to a break in the procedures related to safety.

Reading through the hidden meaning of tattoos, anyone can form a valid opinion about a person tattooed all over.

Many Maya or Aztec symbols are quite popular tattoo graphics for South and Central American criminal gangs, in and out of jails. Some police specialists believe that such hieroglyphs represent numbers which indicate the rank of the wearer. Most such tattoos are executed in black or blue ink, while those in red are reserved for high ranking members such as gang generals or captain.

Since the specific linguistic characteristics of the Mayas or of the Aztecs have been lost over the ages, the Latin American gangs use superstition connotations mixed with Christian faith elements.

That explains the popularity of the "Santa Muerte", (Saint Death"), the "Cuetzpallin",("Lizard"), or the "Coatl", ("Serpent").

They are all, colorful symbols from the past, however they are reminiscent of a period of time when human sacrifices were part of the religious practices. Perhaps that's why the South American gangs are so brutal and blood-thirsty. To a casual observer these criminal gangs seem organized in a random fashion, yet to a specialist they demonstrate a rigid structure which follows the ancient Aztec social structure.

POOR-JUDGMENT TATTOOS

Many individuals, not affiliated in any way with criminal gangs, acquire a large variety of tattoos for reasons hard to explain, except as result of poor judgment. They align along the lines of many fields of human activity, likes and dislikes, opinions, political convictions, or simply for aesthetic "value":

Professional life: they include anchors for mariners, airplanes for pilots, horses and cows for ranchers, fences for Realtors, etc.

Military life: "USMC", "USAF", "US Army, US Navy, rank symbols, etc.

Sports life: Emblems of favorite teams in the NFL, NBA, NHL, etc.:

Hobby preferences: birds, cats, dogs, bicycles, motorcycles, etc.;

Civil social status: "HH",(Head of household), "WW", (Twice widow);

Travel history: Names of the countries visited, tattooed on arms;

Beloved pets: Names of pets tattooed on arms;

Recreational drug users: Marijuana leaves;

Olympic successes: Olympic rings, balls, canoe, tennis rackets, etc.

Medical alerts: Blood type, pacemakers, diabetics, epileptics, etc.

Club affiliations: Lions, Rotarians, Kiwanis, NRA, etc.

Fraternal organizations: Masons, Knights of Columbus, Elks, etc.;

Alma mater emblems: Colleges and universities;

Religious emblems: Cross, Star of David, Star and Crescent, etc.;

Pride in cities: Chicago, I love NY, etc.

Many populations, in Alaska and in Canada use tattooing as a means to record memorable family or clan events. That includes births, deaths, marriages, or devastating natural phenomena, like earthquakes, avalanches or floods.

The graphic characteristics of such tattoos are quite simple: only dots, lines, or semicircles. That was used by the old people living in the arctic regions. The new generations, however, due to alcoholism and to drug abuse get to spend a lot of time in jail, where they get exposed to jailhouse art manifested through some tattoos which are foreign to their culture. That's why one can find a lot of Inuit, Yupik, Alutiiq, or Cupik people, in Alaska or Canada sporting tattoos with images typically of European or Oriental origin.

Before of the turn of the century, in 1890s, the custom of tattooing women disappeared completely, and the men only did tattoo certain parts of their bodies, but rarely their faces.

The Orthodox Church in Alaska and in Canada started a drive to discourage tattooing in the Eskimo communities, after some traveling tattoo artists spread diseases among the people they tattooed, and the health authorities stepped in to stop that practice.

A principal factor that deterred tattooing in the arctic regions was the fact the Eskimos covered all their bodies with heavy cloths capable to protect them in sub-zero temperatures, and there was no way to display any tattoos.

Consequently, the only places youngsters could get tattoos, were in jails, getting rid of any justification that tattoos may show an elevated social status.

The following examples illustrate unequivocally the social status elements of the wearer:

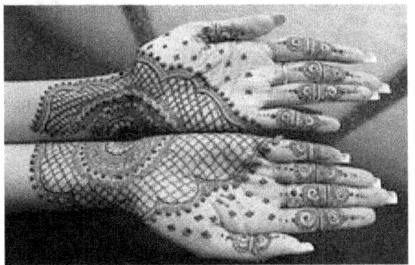

Tattoos on the palms of a noble Indian lady.

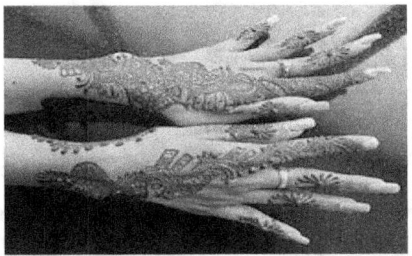

Tattoos on the hands of a noble Indian lady.

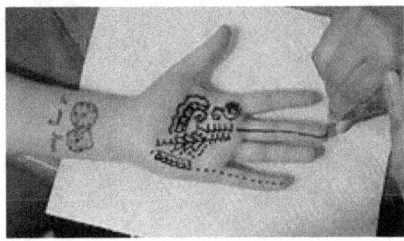

Indian tattoos indicating social cast.

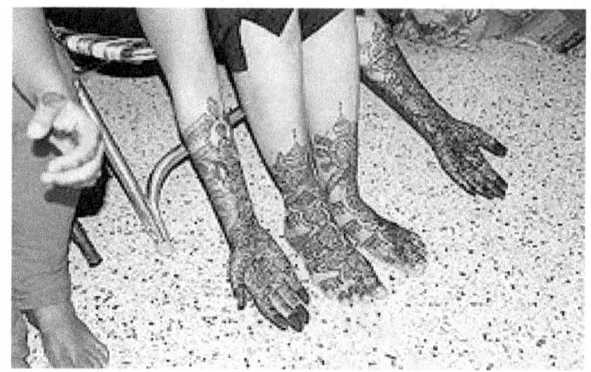

Tattoos on the hands and feet of an Indian wedding party

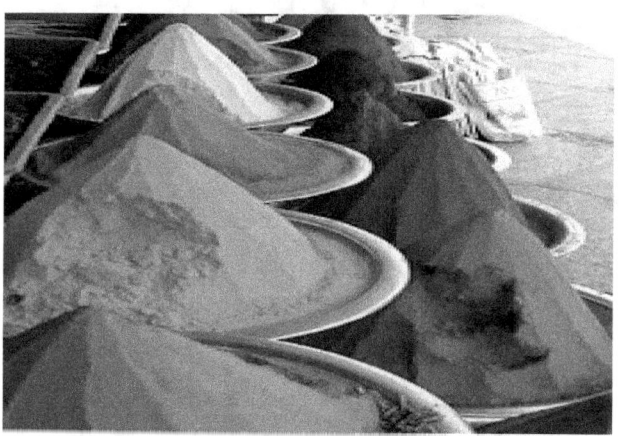

These Kum-Kum powders used for tattoo inks.

The inks and dyes used to tattoo people have various origins. The most widely used materials are the Kum-Kum powders, produced in India, and were widely used there, for millennia, for important religious and social reasons.

Most tattoo powders are made from turmeric which mixed with calcium hydroxide, $Ca(OH)_2$, will turn the yellow turmeric powder into a vivid red. Many types of modern religions are based on a paganism of naturalistic and eco-centric origin, and are heavily supported by leftist ideologies. Some of these Pagans cultivate their beliefs and practices as a form of religious naturalism, copying the behavior of simple forms of life. They practice the tattooing as a way to set their groups apart from the "uninitiated". These groups consider themselves as the pure religious naturalists, and thrive on the so called "Humanistic Paganism", by purveying all sorts of nature-centered views which seem quite offensive to many other religions.

They promote heavy tattooing as a means to assert their "superior" status. The graphics of their tattoos copy the outlines of "living things", differentiating all of them into basic elements belonging to the "Animal Regnum", "Vegetal Regnum", or to the "Mineral Regnum". They deny the existence of the soul, and view the human beings as inferior forms of life. Most of their theoretical religious instruction sessions will not allow the pronunciation of the word "God".

Some of the members of such Humanistic Paganism cults practice tattooing in order to establish and promote their hierarchal order of the membership, into Bishops, Priests, Worshipers and Novices.

Many of the more affluent members of their communities take frequent trips to Africa, Asia and Oceania, where they would photograph tattoos displayed by the local people, in order to copy them for the voluntary use of any "parishioners".

At times, tattoo artists who get such images originated in the far corners of the globe, will incorporate them in the graphics they offer to their clientele. On such an occasion, an American sailor was assaulted by some Samoan people who pointed to his tattoos: "This is the man who likes the spirit who killed Malietoa!". Malietoa was, obviously, a venerated folk hero who died fighting the evil of foreign occupiers. His tattoos proclaimed, in unequivocal terms, some horrible historical facts that our man did could not know.

The author is aware of a case in which a group of Marines on leave in Japan, after consuming a lot of sake, got into a Tokyo tattoo parlor and ordered some fancy graphics. One of the young men, waiting his turn to be tattooed, fell soundly asleep, and his buddies dragged him on the tattoo table where, at his friends' insistence the artist tattooed on his back, in large red letters, "Stupid". His friends could not stop laughing on their way back to the hotel, while the new tattoo owner, had no idea why. Some several months later he discovered what the tattoo on his back was all about. After discharge from the military, upon return to the USA, he had to have that tattoo removed at an exorbitant cost. And finally, after spending a lot of money, and enduring the pain that went with that operation, he was able to go to the beach again.

This is a classic example of how an involuntary tattoo can be placed upon a totally "innocent" person.

The ubiquitous image of the skull and bones, first used by the pirates, found its way into the criminal gangs, and in the academic circles, at the same time. Fraternities at notable universities in the USA claim copyright privileges for the very same symbol.

Similar coincidences regarding "ownership" of tattoo graphics are not too common. There is only one judicial precedent in which a tattoo artist, in California, claimed infringement on his "intellectual property rights", by another person who used his proprietary templates. The case was settled with some small civil compensation to the original author, in 1999.

RELIGIOUS TATTOOS

In Asia, followers of certain religions are obligated to have specific marks on their forehead, made with inks derived from turmeric (Kum-Kum) plants:

The followers of Siva: apply three white horizontal lines with a central dot;

The followers of Vishnu: use two vertical lines, intersected by a red streak;

The followers of the Swaminaraya faith: use one dot at the center of the forehead, most likely in black, but also in red, outside India.

Some Gypsy gangs in Europe, and USA, force their young females to have a red dot tattooed at the center of their foreheads.

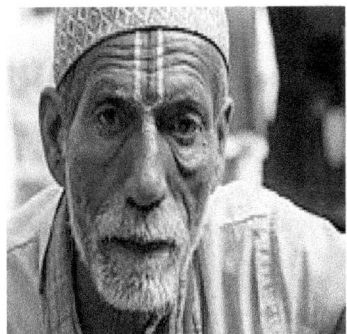 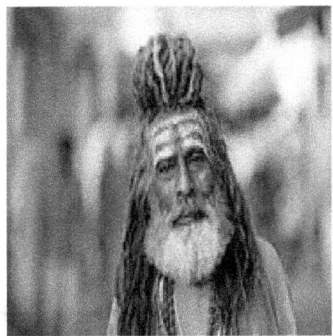

Hindu religious tattoos

The Hindus do not consider themselves "pagans", yet various pagan cults, in America and Europe, adopt their symbolism and translate it into tattoo images with several hidden meanings, that baffle researchers.

Chinese followers of the Kung Fu, (Confucius), philosophy, will wear tattoos proclaiming ancient wisdom sayings, and practical teachings regarding leadership, commerce, morals, and astronomy.

Religious pagan tattoo symbols

To an uninitiated person, many of such symbols may look just like the branding symbols, used in marking herds of cattle in Texas or other Southwestern states. It seems that the preferred color is black, but there is no explanation for that.

Some of the most notorious gang members use their own "religious" symbols animated by superstition, and not by a belief in God, or in any recognizable religion.

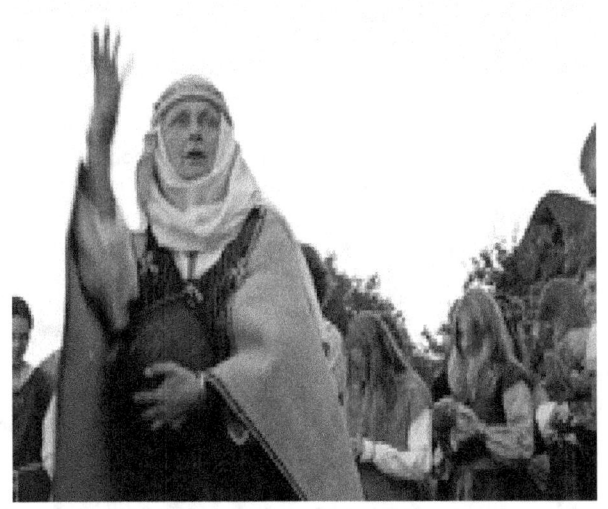

Pagan naturalist priestess preaching in Northern California (1964)

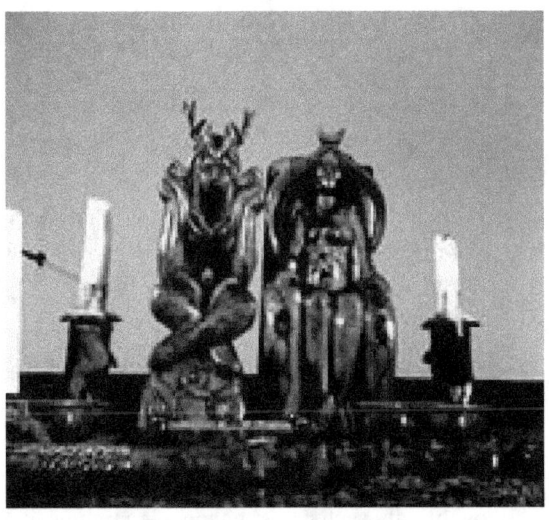

Charles Manson's pagan altar

One of the most repulsive pagan movements in the Western USA was that started by Charles Manson crime family. It popularized the idea that the Swastika has a concentrated "spiritual power", which constantly needs new human blood to survive, and to empower certain followers to survive adversity.

This particular crime group advocated indiscriminate sex with all of the females, claiming that this way the "animal power" would manifest itself like some sort of animal spirit, protecting and helping all the "family" members.

During wild sessions of community sex, Charles Manson preached about the sexual duality, like a divine sort of alternate spirit, justifying both heterosexuality and homosexuality. The horrible crimes committed by his adherents were fully "justified" by the need to spill the blood of the inferior animals. Certain human beings were included in this category.

For that reason Charles Manson had a swastika tattooed on his forehead while his followers had swastikas tattooed on other body parts.

This cult plagiarized some lyrical elements from the then-contemporary music, claiming ownership, and selling such albums as original music. Their followers delighted in spreading such tunes, even though the central idea in every song was the need to murder "unworthy people".

The tattoos worn by Charles Manson followers expressed the idea of the coming racial war to purify the mankind, and the acute "necessity" to wash it in the blood of the enemies of the "family", meaning actually against social harmony.

The leader of this crime family insisted that all his followers wear recognition tattoos, which, supposedly, had a spiritual power to protect and to grant success in everything they do.

No one knows for sure why so many people in that group did follow blindly such a misfit and an ignoramus like Charles Manson.

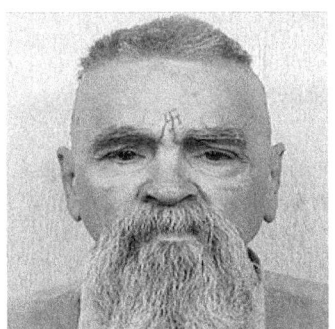

Charles Manson's swastika tattoo

As a vicious White Supremacist, Charles Manson hoped to ignite an all-out race war, in which Blacks, Hispanics, Jews, and immigrants would be totally eliminated. That did not occur until the first 20 years of the 21st century, when violent race manifestations appeared to be motivated by certain political events.

In Charlottesville, VA, as an example, white supremacists clashed with leftist counter-demonstrators, resulting in severe injuries and one death. The local police was not able to separate the two fighting mobs. Moreover, a local police official was quoted as telling the police force to: "Stand down and let them kill each other…"

And to think that the right of free speech would be protected by the US Constitution seems to be a fallacy, no matter what political flavor was used! Charles Manson and his followers rejected the idea that they were part of a religious cult, yet they constantly preached from the position of a Doomsday Cult missionary, with the aim to incite a race war that would "purify" the world, by eliminating any of the "unworthy nations", aka Blacks, Hispanic, Jews, Catholics, immigrants, and Orientals.

While in prison, the Manson family followed with attention all the news, and concluded that their dreams were just about to materialize in a racial war, especially after the Los Angeles and Chicago events of 1964. When studying gangs and cults, like that just described, it can be safely assumed that lack of religion can be considered, in itself, a religion!

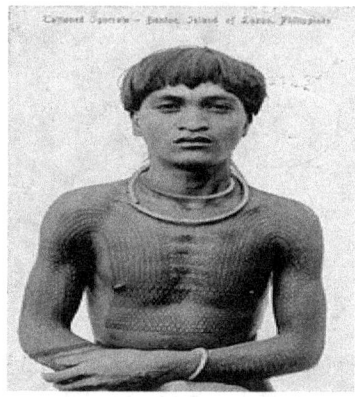

Tattoos on the body of a Filipino headhunter (1850)

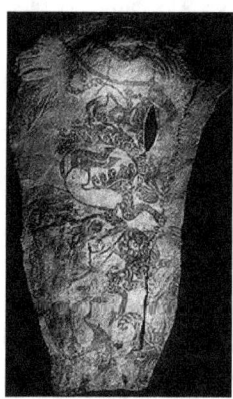

Tattoos on the arm of a mummy, circa 3,000 BC

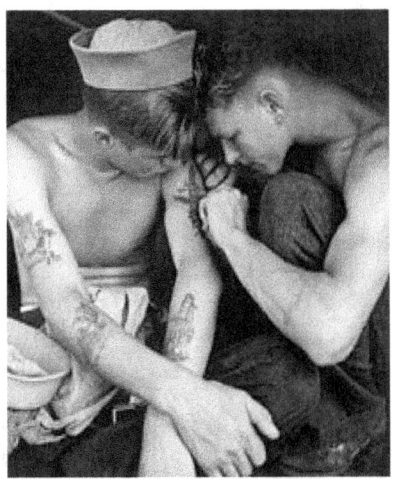

US sailors getting tattoos on board of USS New Jersey (1949)

No one can argue that the oldest tattoos ever found on Egyptian mummies, do not have any religious connotations. They wanted to get divine protection while revealing their social status, as nobles, or extremely rich people, most likely, as generals, or as high-ranking soldiers. If one examines tattoo graphics over the years, the history of the human race emerges clearly, almost like in a documentary.

The range of subject matter covered by tattoo graphics encompasses absolutely every single possible social position, more so on the outskirts of larger cities with masses of uneducated, poor people.

The tattooing of those people indicates, quite significantly, a transition from a low economic class, to adherence to criminal gangs displaying a lot of material progress, by the clothes they wear, and the vehicles they drive. They are well-armed with weapons which often are better than those used by the law enforcement personnel.

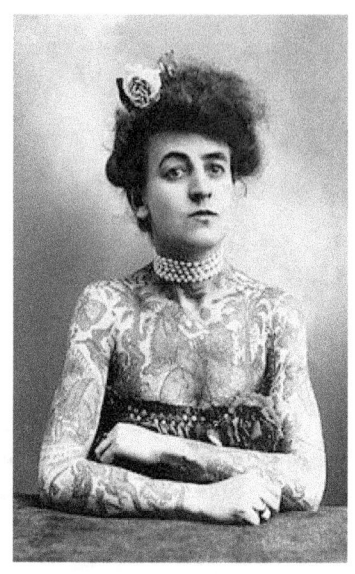

American Gypsy circus performer (1917)

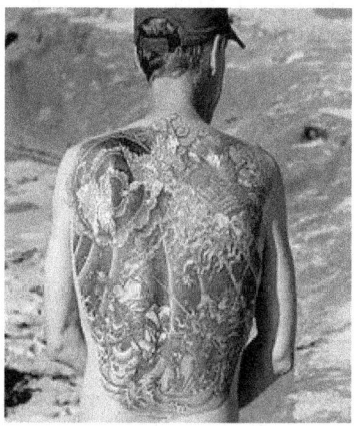

Hippie tattoo art (1965)

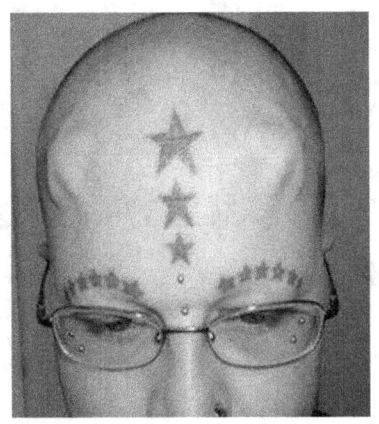

"Intellectual" tattoo (2002)

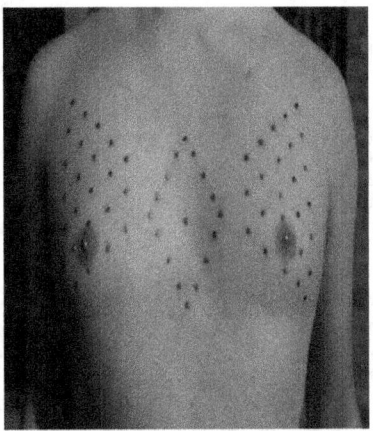

Tattoo made through burning (2001)

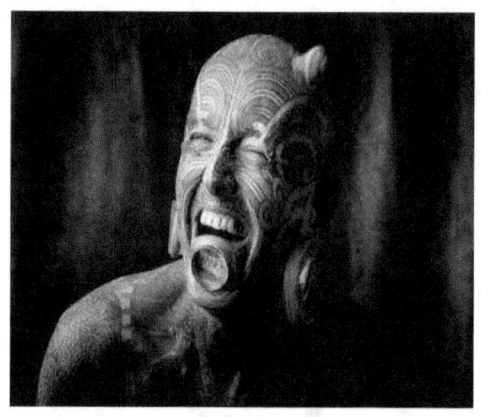

Extreme tattooing with mutilation (1979)

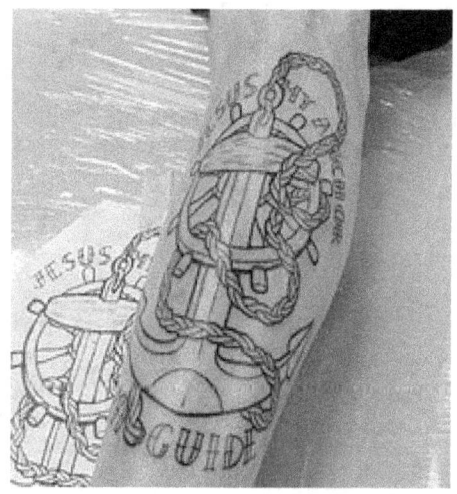

Typical sailor tattoo next to the artist's template

THE MUSLIM BROTHERHOOD

Also known as the "Society of the Muslim Brothers" was founded in 1928 in Egypt by the Islamic scholar Hassan el-Banna, as a full theocratic political organization, with wide populist support in the Arab world. Initially this organization excelled in charity work, but in the 1950s it took an aggressive stance against "non-believers", notably against Israel and the USA. Consequently it accepted the idea of religious justification for political assassinates, as a tool for achieving a holy common goal. Saddam Hussein, and other Muslim leaders gained power through political killings approved and applauded by a score of religious Islamic leaders.

This organization was the heart and soul of the "Arab spring" in 2011 which caused the fall of several governments in Africa, (Egypt and Libya), however, a lot of the neighboring Arab governments considered it just a terrorist organization.

So did the USA, Russia, EU, UK, Bahrain, Syria, Saudi Arabia, the United Arab Emirates, and Israel. Oddly enough, Iran, with a Shiite theocracy form of government, does not support this Islamic movement, because it was founded by Sunni Islamists.

As a matter of fact, the Iranian government imprisoned hundreds of members of the Iranian Muslim Brotherhood. Many countries started a hard crackdown on all Muslim Brotherhood members, for alleged terrorist activities.

The texts tattooed on the arms of the Muslim Brotherhood members normally read, in classic Arabic: "There is no God but Allah". It was reported that President Barack Obama wore a ring with the same inscription, on his left hand, the closes to his heart.

The author was unable to verify this fact, which many people would attribute to hate toward a Black president as a practicing Muslim.

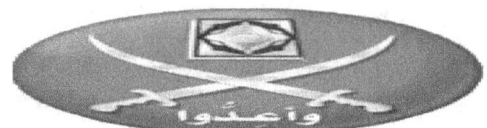

Muslim Brotherhood tattoo (1960). The text reads in in Arabic: "There is no God, but Allah, the all-powerful".

Even though Muslim scholars preach against tattooing, many members of the Society of Muslim Brothers may have some multiple tattoos on their arms and chests, with specific symbolism, including quotes from the Koran, or images representing either the flags of the "Future World Caliphate", or of their countries of birth, or coats of arms with a crescent and a star, not much unlike some of the official flags of several Muslim countries.

Some journalists alleged that President Barack Obama, was an active member of the Muslim Brotherhood, ever since his days in Indonesia, under the guidance of his stepfather. They based these accusations on the fact that he was wearing a gold ring on his left hand with the Arabic inscription "No God but Allah". They also observed that during Ramadan Barack Obama did not wear his jewelry, since the practicing Muslims are commanded to be modest, and not to wear any jewelry during that holiday. At any rate, in his speeches to Muslim audiences, the US President Barack Hussein Obama II took the ideological position of the Muslim Brotherhood, in blaming USA for all the ills that plagued the Islamic society, apologizing for that situation.

The same journalists followed that president on the sandy beaches of Hawaii, to ascertain if he had any tattoos that could raise some other issues along the same allegations. The results were negative.

They could not discover any tattoos on the body of Barack Obama. Most of the controversial issues triggered by the frequent investigations into the circumstances of his birth, religious affiliation, and in his parental origin, were tied to some Kenyan people, were put to rest, by unequivocal declarations made by the next US president, Donald J. Trump, during his electoral campaign in 2016.

Nevertheless, a large segment of the Muslim people, both in the USA and outside, continue to maintain a toxic attitude toward the US President, accusing him of being an anti-Islamist, and a lot of other sins, when, in fact, as the commander-in-chief the President was charged with the country's protection against the radical Muslim terrorism.

The Muslim Brotherhood is the original incubator for a lot of toxic terrorist organizations which will not abstain from anything in order to reach their goals of total world domination. The list of organizations considered as offshoots of the Muslim Brotherhood includes names that read just like the "Who's Who" in the criminal world, due to their actions: murder, kidnappings, rape, torture, etc.

The following Muslim organizations, all inspired, and mentored by the original Muslim Brotherhood, are powerful criminal gangs, who practice religious and anti-social terrorism, all over the world, dead set to blow Israel off the map of the world, and to destroy the USA.

They consider the USA the "Great Satan" that Allah will ultimately conquer. The main terrorist offshoots are:

Abu Sayyaf, which as a paramilitary Islamic organization, of Wahhabi jihad- type ideology, operates in the Philippines, Brazil, Iraq, and in Mexico, where they participate in the drug trade. They number less than 5,000 members, and like to use improvised explosives, mortars, and assault rifles, to kill people they consider inferior nonbelievers.

Al-Itihaad al-Islamiya, ("The Islamic Union"), is an Islamic terrorist group started in Somalia, in early 1990. It professes total hatred toward all nonbelievers, and gets its money from kidnappings and from mercenary formations in service to local warlords. It is estimated to have some 2,000 followers.

Al Shabaab, or "Youth Movement", is a jihadist Islamic terror group, , started in East Africa in early 1990s. It is notorious for their degree of savagery in torturing and beheading their prisoners. They number around 10,000 members, but international pressure determined their leadership to order most of their "troops" to leave urban areas in favor of remote rural settings. They recruited heavily from Central African nations, and executed all the recruits who had tattoos. Their preferred methods of action are hijackings of trucks, arms contraband, kidnapping of foreigner females, which are sold as slaves. This terrorist group claims "ancient" tribal rights over the entire country of Ethiopia, and have assassinated savagely more than five thousand Ethiopian Christians.

Boko Haram is a group of Western African terrorist organizations which displays a strict Islamic ideology – "Haram" refers to all the elements interdicted by the Koran, like certain food or western customs. It was started in 2000 in Nigeria, and is active in Chad, Nigeria, Cameroon, and Congo, counting on some more than 10,000 "Soldiers of Islam". They forbid western education under the penalty of death, and extract steep "taxes" from all people who do not pledge their families and businesses to this group. They are notorious for piracy, kidnappings, extortion, and bombings, which result in hundreds of innocent victims. They execute all the new recruits to have their arms tattooed.

Dar al Islam, meaning the "Islamic Armed Forces", was started in Indonesia in early 1940s, and at this time it numbers over 20,000 guerilla troops, spread all over the country. They derive their income primarily through criminal enterprises which include, kidnappings, slavery, illegal gambling, (not permitted by the Koran), and extortion of companies owned by foreigners, even if they are Muslims. They have a total prohibition for tattoos, in order to prevent member detection.

Gerakan Mujahadin, or the "Pattani Islamiya al-Gerakan Mujahadin", (The right-belief fighters) is a small terrorist gang, operating in southern Indonesia and Malaysia. This group was established in the early 2000s, and numbers less than 3000 members, but is notorious for blowing up venues frequented by foreign tourists. They all sport tattoos with Koran quotes, but no one can tell exactly how they derive the money needed to buy arms and explosives. Their leaders use only pseudonyms, a fact that baffle the local police.

Hamas, ("Courage"), or the "Resistance Movement", is an Islamic Sunni criminal gang originated in the areas of Gaza, Egypt, Jordan and Iraq, with the only goal to destroy Israel, and the western culture. Founded in the early 1980s, today it numbers over 50,000 "soldiers", who constantly kill Israeli civilians and western travelers. Its money comes from Iran, Saudi Arabia and United States. While Hillary Clinton was US Secretary of State, under the Obama administration, she granted Hamas over 150 million dollars for "cultural works", which ended up as rockets and bullets shot at Israel.

Hamas is opposed to any peaceful solution of the Israeli-Arab conflict, frequently attacking PLO officials, and insists adamantly that all Arabs have the obligation to kill Jews. Current polls in the area show that most Arabs want peace, and dissociate from Hamas.

Hezbollah, or the "Party of Allah", is a Shi'a Islamist terrorist group financed largely by Iran, and was founded in Lebanon in the early 1980s. Its main objectives are the total destruction of Israel, and of the royal family of Saudi Arabia. There are over 20,000 Hezbollah members, throughout the Arab countries, out of which some over 1,000 are in Israeli jails. Hezbollah negotiates frequent prisoner exchanges with Israel, under a formula of approximately three terrorists for each IDF soldier. This terrorist group does not allow tattoos on "God's soldiers" and is not too concerned with raising money. All they want to do is to instill "God's fear" and panic among all the

Israeli civilians. They use bombings, shootings, disinformation campaigns. Hezbollah sent a contingent of some 5,000 fighters, in 1993, to fight the Serbian Christians in Bosnia. Most Sunni Muslims in Lebanon oppose the Hezbollah's agenda and the Saudi Arabian royal family regards their guerilla tactics as un-Islamic, calling them "terrorists".

Taliban, ("Students" in Pashtoon), is the terrorist Islamic organization which absorbed the Al Qaeda, ("The Base"), the Bin Laden's brainchild in Afghanistan, as an insurrection formation, with over 100,000 "soldiers". In early 1996 it emerged as one of the primary factions in the Afghan Civil War, gaining a considerable land area, controlling it through improvised explosive devices, mortar fire, and assassinations of local people perceived as "traitors".

The Taliban obtains a large amount of income through the opium trade, estimated to be over three million dollars per month. That's how they can purchase modern armament to "Punish the enemies of Allah", who invaded their country.

As a basic Sunni Islamic fundamentalist movement, the Taliban benefits of material support from Saudi Arabia, Pakistan, and from the American Muslims. Recently, they suffered serious losses against the Karzai administration, and the NATO-led coalition of the International Security Assistance Forces. Sadly enough, after more than 15 years of war, the prospects of peace are nowhere in sight. After the capture and killing of Osama Bin Laden, the Taliban moved its base of operations to Pakistan, where they use successfully suicide bombers, often disguised as local police, extracting a heavy toll of casualties from the civilian population

The Taliban use various, tried guerilla methods, to terrorize the population, and the foreign "invaders", primarily through surprise IED bombings, suicide missions, mortar attacks, kidnappings, and assassinations of local administrative leaders.

The Taliban have been condemned internationally, for their obtuse interpretation of the Koran, in the Sharia courts, especially in regard to the treatment of women.

In five years of Taliban rule, from 1996 to 2001, over 100,000 people were savagely massacred, thousands of homes destroyed, and by practicing a method of "scorched earth" warfare, they denied livelihood to a whole agrarian society.

Hisbul Islamyia, ("The Islamic Party"), is a Somali insurgent group formed in 2005, in Mogadishu, after which some half of its 10,000 members merged with the older Al Shabaab Islamic terrorist group. The practices and the aims of this group are very much similar to those used by the Taliban in Afghanistan and Pakistan, except for the fact that they lack the technical sophistication of their members, and many of their acts end up in total fiasco. As an example, in 2015 they tried to assassinate a local warlord, Sharif Sheik Ahmed, the leader of the Harti clan, and the ten-man team tasked with that operation perished in a premature explosion, leveling two city blocks in Mogadishu. Sheik Ahmed was trying to build a coalition to end the lawlessness there. Most all the activities of this group, includes a minority aligned with Al Shabaab, but now, it fights against it, and against the central government, using the theme of the Second Civil War in Somalia, for the "re-liberation" of the country. That civil war continues to rage since 2009.

Since Hisbul Islamyia was pushed away as a major combatant, and was relegated to a very small area, in the sparsely-populated Southern Somalia, they continue with brazen acts of piracy, and horrible kidnappings for ransom, mostly against UN personnel delivering food and medical aid.

Sharif Sheik Ahmed, an intellectual educated in Egypt and Libya, issued several orders prohibiting tattooing of its forces, which was thus interpreted by many, as a hostile act directed against the African traditions, fact which attracted opposition to his movement. He survived however, several attempts to be assassinated.

The drive to establish a provisional government in Somalia, capable to curb the anarchy and the lawlessness which plagued this country for over 30 years, was torpedoed by the same terrorist organization founded by the Sharif Sheik Ahmed.

One of the main characteristics of most all Muslim terrorist groups consists in a type of fluidity, which constantly changes allegiances, in spite of the fact that all of them claim to have some sort of monopoly on the "True Islam".

This type of changes makes the job of those who study them, quite difficult.

The claims made by most all Islamic terrorist groups, that they are interested in the welfare of all their subjects, by founding charity and assistance programs, are totally baseless. The hunger is the only element that is common in Africa, in all the territories controlled by these violent Islamic movements, especially in those conquered by the "true Islamists".

The only common denominator of the life under the rule of such groups is terror, hunger, disease, and a total lack of elementary items of modern conveniences, like clean drinking water, electrical energy and medical assistance.

That explains the horrible mortality rate of infants, and the extremely short life span of all people living under the rules of the Islamic insurgent groups.

It seems that the interpretation of the Koran is frequently perverted by people with no religious education, simply as a fast way to the absolute power.

Boko Haram, Allahia, (Boko haram for Allah),moved from hitting soft targets, like mosques, schools, soccer games, and bus stations, to bombing United Nation facilities, set up to provide food and medical assistance to the millions of people needing it.

Spreading the ideas that western medicine including all types of vaccines, are a method used by non-believers to kill Muslims, they create animosity and resentment toward those who want to save their lives.

In a horrific ambush in the city of Abuja, in December 2016, upon two UN convoys of trucks carrying food and medicine, Boko Haram for Allah, killed all the 50 UN employees working in Nigeria. Incidentally, they all were Muslims from Egypt.

The cruelty of this group, best known for kidnapping young school girls, became legendary. Out of over 300 little girls just 150 were saved, after being sold as slaves on the slave markets of Nigeria, Cameroon, Biafra and Central Africa.

Please note that slavery is an accepted Islamic practice, regardless affiliation, be it Sunni or Shia. Male slaves may gain freedom by converting to Islam, while women are rarely allowed any kind of choice.

Human trafficking seems to be a very lucrative endeavor for most Muslim gangs, regardless their professed religious or political views.

While discussing the ways in which most gangs make money, we do need to examine also the substance of foreign aid granted by the generous State Department to various Muslim countries in the hope of tempering down the notion of waging war against defenseless populations. Based on this idiotic concept of throwing money at a problem in hope to solve it that way, a lot of US taxpayer dollars end up in the wrong hands. The main idea of helping certain countries, like Tanzania and Nigeria, was motivated by the need to diminish the Chinese influence there, in favor of the US, through agricultural implements meant to rehabilitate a socialist economy.

POLITICAL GANGS

There are political groups that some people call "gangs" since they are just as criminal and as vicious, as the street criminal gangs, or the prison gangs. They may cover a large spectrum of political believes, from the far right to the far left.

The far right political gangs may include the Ku Klux Klan, the Neo-Fascists, the National-Socialists, the Anarchists, and few others. Basically they are anti-social and channel their hate and aggression against certain groups, such as Jews, immigrants, federal employees, etc. They will go as far as to blow up government buildings or to assassinate some politicians they do not like. Timothy McVey, the Oklahoma City bomber, was one of them.

The far left political gangs are represented by Communists, Socialists, Marxists, Black Panthers, Weather Underground, and a few other minor groups just as toxic and lethal as those mentioned above.

They all hate the US Constitution and its provisions, they are utterly anti-American, anti-social, and anti-everything. They refuse to engage in political dialog, preferring to use violence and intimidation to silence any opposition. Beatings and murders are verified methods they use to kill the constitutional freedoms. They consider all their opponents as lower forms of life, thus fit to be exterminated. They preach about racial superiority, regardless whether they are White or Black, and advance the idea that the American society owes them a great deal of "gratitude" for what they do. Since during their demonstrations they wear disguises, such as hoods, capes, masks, etc. it is quite difficult to identify them in order to ascertain the types of tattoos they have. It would be safe to assume that their tattoo graphics include the "hammer and sickle", swastika, stars, crosses, fists, and the single finger. Being loosely-organized in state chapters, they try to avoid exposure to the media scrutiny, except for very rare occasions.

TATTOO REMOVAL

For long periods of time, all the tattoos were considered permanent, almost impossible to remove. Historical events, and some social changes, dictated the need to have some tattoos removed, primarily for the safety of the wearers.

Several primitive methods were used for that, such as rubbing with salt until the entire outer skin was removed with considerable pain. During the 19th century, some physicians had limited success in removing tattoos with chemicals like, tri-chlorine-acetic acid, (TCA), which dissolved the epidermis, all the way to the level in which the tattoo ink or pigment was injected.

Cryosurgery uses liquefied nitrogen, and can yield some good results. Frequently, this method of tattoo removal needed skin grafts, fact which complicated things.

Since the early 1990s after the introduction of the medical lasers, this type of surgical intervention proved effective, with minimal pain. The most frequently used techniques employed in surgical tattoo removal were the "continuous wave lasers", and the intermittent high intensity light pulses.

Using lasers, black or dark inks can be removed almost completely.

When someone needs to get rid of a tattoo, many options may look too troublesome, and the solution is to cover-up the tattoo, with one which can obscure the original one.

An artfully executed second tattoo may render the old one totally invisible, depending on color, size, and specific details. To cover an old tattoo it is necessary to use much darker inks on the new tattoo.

If the old tattoo used too dark inks, a cover-up solution may not work. In such cases a laser treatment is suggested. That way the laser beam would break the ink particles and the body's immune system would reject and eliminate them as foreign matter, exactly just like in the case of fading due to time and sun. Some of the inks, particularly yellow or fluorescent ones, are extremely hard to remove due to low absorption index, which falls outside the envelope of laser energy.

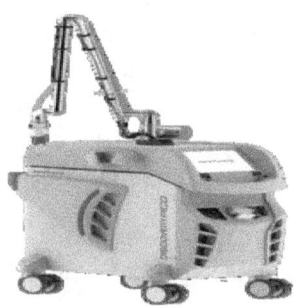

Typical surgical laser used to remove tattoos. (Discovery 2015)

Laser tattoo removal requires topical anesthesia, but the scarring cannot be avoided 100%. That's why most people with tattoos regret the decision to get them.

The normal human growth, causes a healing process which has a tendency to eliminate foreign bodies, however, some of the tattoo pigment particles are too large for that. The laser treatment will heat up, and will break apart all the ink particles into smaller pieces, thus making them susceptible to elimination through normal physiological reactions. The laser pulses will, also, minimize scarring. The main factors affecting the laser treatment efficiency, in tattoo removal, are:

- The color of the laser shall be selected as to penetrate into the skin layer where the tattoo ink was injected;

- The laser energy shall be fully absorbed, in order to heat up and to break ink particles;

- The duration of the laser pulses has to be extremely short, of the order of a few nanoseconds;

- Too high a laser energy level results in scarring, too low a laser energy level, it does not fragment sufficiently the pigment particles.

Pain management, post-treatment factors, together with the side effects and possible complications, need to be thoroughly assessed by the surgeons, in cases in which multiple laser sessions are necessary.

Even if the laser treatments to remove tattoos are common procedures, there are certain factors which invite caution. Some people, most likely with dark skin, may develop hypopigmentation, changing the color and the texture of the skin into lighter tones.

The patients with light-tone skin, with blonde or red hair, may experience a hyperpigmentation which causes dark skin spots.

Since some pigments contain metallic powders, the laser action may induce a wider distribution of ink particles in the body, causing unexpected toxicity. Laser removal of certain tattoos has been reported to cause the ignition of many inks which contained chemicals similar to those used in fireworks.

The process of removing tattoos with lasers, causes ulcerations on the epidermis, dermis, and on the subcutaneous tissues. That may trigger severe infections, or gangrene, if not properly diagnosed and treated. A regimen of antibiotics, judiciously selected, would take care of such side effects. One of the most prevalent side effects in tattoo removal is generated by skin infections, and skin neoplasms, or skin cancer. There is a whole list of skin pathogenic conditions, associated with the art of tattooing, or with tattoo removal: patches, papule, plaque, nodules, cysts, tumors, fissures, ulcers, eczema, and the atrophy of portions of tissue, etc. Of course, the determining factor in ascertaining all the risk factors related to tattooing, or tattoo removal, is the general state of the patient's health, his or her fitness from a point of view regarding the immune system.

Any physiological problems, along these lines, may result in more severe problems, rarely commensurate with any of the benefits derived from tattoo removal.

This simply demonstrates that when it comes to human body, there is no action without a reaction. Some times this relation is quite unexpected, since there are so many variables that have to be taken into account. An experienced surgeon would handle this type of situation properly, mitigating the proportionality between risk factors versus benefits.

In conclusion, it is interesting to observe that a tattoo made in a hurry, without proper thinking beforehand, can induce some dire consequences that a wearer may regret for a long time.

Unsuccessful tattoo removal would provide a person the same "benefits" he or she got when first obtained the tattoo.

- A severe limitation in options for a better life,

- A certain stigma, caused by the inability to join some social circles, like country clubs, academic achievement classifications, etc.

- An extremely critical view of all kinds of work performed by anyone with visible tattoos;

- The mistaken assumption that a tattoo would symbolize an important life achievement;

- Doubt about the character and professionalism of the wearer if the only remained part of the original tattoo is a scar.

But again, this is life! All the mistakes have to be repaid in full.

No one shall argue about the "importance" of any "original" tattoo. The position that this is some sort of fashion accessory, or a declaration of social status, may work well in sub-Sahara Africa or in Oceania, but here, in the USA is just a fallacy. Aside from religious considerations, a tattoo is still a proof of primitivism, especially in the age when the human race just did step up to a type two civilization, when it became possible, due to technological advances, to leave the planet. Like many other things considered "artistic", the "beauty" of any tattoo remains in the eyes of the beholder, just like the graffiti on a national monument.

The psychological elements related to the "buyer's remorse", after acquiring a tattoo, may not be immediately apparent, however, after a certain period of time they become significant.

Studies in this sense revealed that over 90% of suicide acts are committed by people with tattoos, and that includes several people with celebrity status, like Ernest Hemingway. Many suicides of people with outstanding social status, have inspired many copy-cat suicides.

Examples of celebrities whose suicides have triggered suicide clusters include the Chinese actor, Ruan Lingyu, the Japanese artists Yukiko Okada, Miyu Uehara, and Chung Lee, the South Korean actress Choi Jin-Sil, whose suicide caused all suicide rates to rise by 162.3% and Marilyn Monroe, whose death was followed by an increase of 200 more suicides than average for that August month. Another famous case is the self-immolation of Mohammed Bouazizi, a Tunisian street vendor, who set himself on fire on December 17, 2010, an act that was a catalyst for the Tunisian Revolution and sparked the Arab Spring which caused several men to emulate Bouazizi's act. A 2017 study published in JAMA Internal medicine magazine, published online the 13 Reasons, which chronicled a fictional teen's suicide was associated with an increase in suicide related Internet searches, including a 26% increase in searches for "how to commit suicide", a 18% increase for "commit suicide" and 9% increase for "how to kill yourself." These findings suggest that copycat suicides might also be connected to the perception that a suicide is a uniquely gratifying experience.

Due to some high-profile suicides, the demand for the same tattoos, as those worn by the celebrity suicide victims, increased almost exponentially during the same month of the media reports. Some bad things seem contagious.

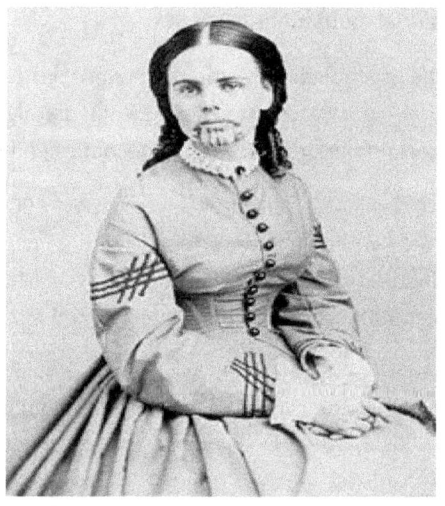

Tattooed lady who committed suicide

EPILOGUE

Most decisions to get tattoos are made on the spur of the moment, and the benefits of such "artistic" endeavors are, always, questionable. The wearers of tattoos realize, often too late, that there may be a serious stigma attached to having them.

That's why a tattoo is considered a voluntary mutilation, where the benefits of the symbolic aspects of the graphic contents are of negative importance, unless certain circumstances dictate that, like in jails, and in criminal street gangs.

Decoding some of the hidden meaning of most tattoo styles, as this booklet attempts to do, is a necessity for police personnel, for managers, and anyone who does the hiring, regardless the size of the organization.

It is much better to avoid hiring a person who would, most likely, jeopardize company assets, as being suggested by tattoos that advertise anti-social behavior.

Aside from the fact that tattoos, in general, demonstrate lack of sound judgment, they place the wearer in the shade of the anti-culture. If the argument of protest against income inequity is used, please observe that it is a law of natural economics, to have unequal income, for unequal efforts, no matter what the tattoo graphics try to demonstrate.

The only thing that tattoos may enforce is the extra tenacity a wearer has to deal with in overcoming all sorts of adversities resulted from stigma. Most people do not want to accept oddities, and that extends to tattoos, studs, or earrings for men, etc.

Those body modifications, or mutilations, go against the elementary Christian tenets, as tantamount to graffiti on God's temple, since the Bible specifies, in more than one place, the fact that the human body has to be considered a temple and a miracle of divine creation. In fact, the Jews and the Catholics are prohibited from getting tattoos, based on the Leviticus 19 text, even though some think that this only applies to the Jews. Learned people claim that there are no rules in the New Testament that will prohibit any tattoos, and most Christian denominations will consider the laws spelled in Leviticus to be outdates. Tattoos are tolerated however, by Evangelical and Fundamental Protestants, yet they believe to be a sin to get one. Coptic Christians in Egypt and Ethiopia tattoo crosses on their right hand as a means of differentiation from Muslims.

Sunni Islam prohibits tattoos as "haram", (not permitted), based on Hadith and various scholarly rulings.

In Shia Islam tattoos are permitted, provided that the imagery and the texts are not offensive to the core beliefs of the community. If they are, then the men wearing them can be severely punished for blasphemy.

Historically, tattooing, (practiced in Egypt for millennia), was considered pagan, and it was prohibited by the Council of Nicaea in 325 AD, even though Roman soldiers were required, at one time, to have their hands tattooed to identify the bodies of those killed in battle, and to make desertion difficult. Emperor Constantine the Great, (272 – 337 AD) prohibited all tattooing among Roman soldiers and officials, under a strict code of conduct based on Roman custom.

Parliamentary protocols, in many countries prohibit the display of visible tattoos during official work sessions. Same rules apply to the members of the executive corps in most international companies, as a requirement included with the dress code.

A visible tattoo is not allowed anywhere in official places.

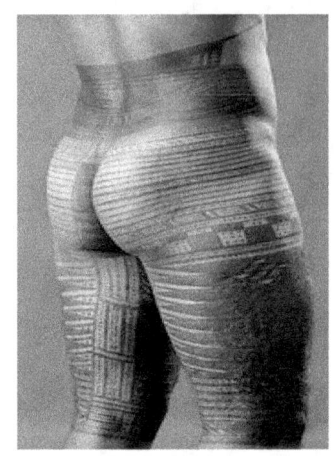

Typical Samoa tattoo (1965)

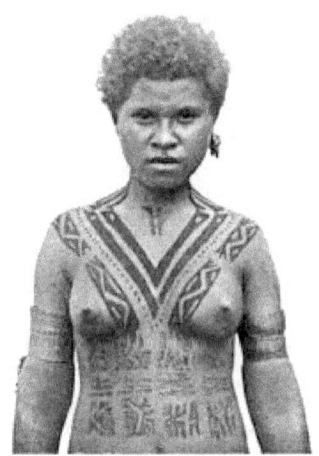

Woman from New Guinea (1976)

No matter how one looks at the tattooing, some questions may seem to pop up when people are exposed to the various styles and graphics used today:

> "Is that person, wearing all those tattoos, a jail bird?"
>
> "Is that person a street criminal gang member?"
>
> "Is that person demonstrating the extent of his or her poor judgment?"

Of course a correct answer is quite difficult to ascertain, especially among the female members of the "Generation X" or "Generation Y"

Aside from the claim to be modern "fashion accessories", the tattooing exposes the people getting them, to grave risk of diseases, such as AIDS, TB, Hepatitis C, staph, various types of Herpes, tetanus, etc. especially in an unsanitary environment, such as that found on the street, or in a jails, where proper medical supervision is not available. The very existence of risk factors is greatly reduced under the category of licensed professional tattoo parlors.

The decision to get a tattoo is a questionable one, if voluntary. Involuntary, tattoos, however, would underline some of the exceptional circumstances, like those found in jails, criminal gangs, or concentration camps.

Contemporary tattoo artists use latex gloves, sterile needles in the tattoo machines, and, generally, follow the recommended sanitary protocols. That reduces considerably the chances of complications due to the transmission of the pathogenic agents, which may contaminate some of the affected skin areas.

No matter what type of tattoo one selects, some risk factors cannot be totally eliminated, since infections may appear outside the controlled area of a tattoo parlor.

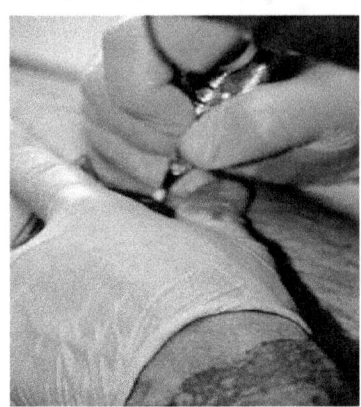

Modern tattoo artist at work (2009)

If the tattooing can be considered "modern art", or a new, radical "fashion statement" the thought that its origins may be found two or three millennia ago then your perspective may change very little. If the process of tattooing was OK for primitive populations and for ancient Egyptians, why not use the same reasoning today?

Similarly to a painter, the tattoo artist uses the human skin as a canvas, and the only limiting factors are offered by the imagination of the artist, and that of his or her client. The aesthetic value of this kind of art remains in the eyes of the beholder. This fact will raise the subjectivism level of such an endeavor, to areas that the ancient populations did not have anything else to compare to. The proud owner of a brand new tattoo, in Africa, would feel the same compulsion to display it fully, expecting admiration, just like a young man in the USA, getting to fulfill a certain psychological need to place himself apart from his pears. There have been scores of studies about the psychological effects of tattoos, including an analysis of obscure merits, which tried to justify the tattoo practice as a need of self-expression for sex appeal. How many people would select a spouse based solely on the aspect of tattoos?

More examples of extreme tattooing;

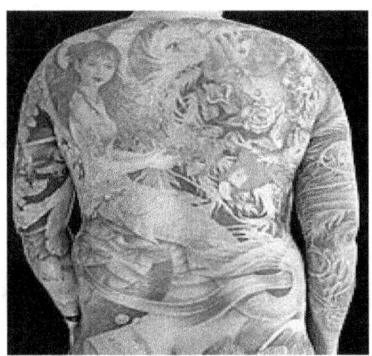

Japanese Sumo wrestlers. (1972)

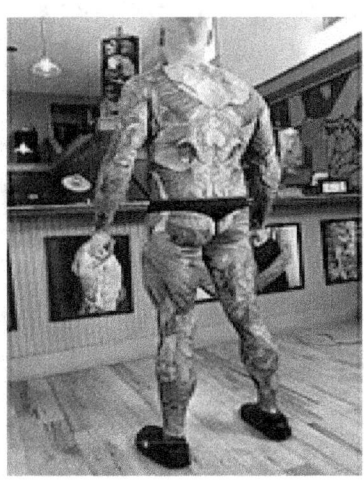

BIBLIOGRAPHY

Buckland, A. W. (1887) "On Tattooing", in *Journal of the Royal Anthropological Institute of Great Britain and Ireland*, 1887/12, p. 318–328

Caplan, Jane (ed.) (2000): *Written on the Body: the Tattoo in European and American History*, Princeton University Press

DeMello, Margo (2000) *Bodies of Inscription: a Cultural History of the Modern Tattoo Community*, California. Durham NC: Duke University Press

Fisher, Jill A (2002). "Tattooing the Body, Marking Culture". Tattoos & Society

Gell, Alfred (1993) *Wrapping in Images: Tattooing in Polynesia*, Oxford:
Gilbert, Stephen G. (2001) *Tattoo History: a Source Book*, New York: Juno Books

Gustafson, Mark (1997) "*Inscripta in fronte*: Penal Tattooing in Late Antiquity", in *Classical Antiquity*, April 1997, Vol. 16/No. 1, p. 79–105

Hambly, Wilfrid Dyson (1925) *The History of Tattooing and Its Significance: With Some*

Hesselt van Dinter, Maarten (2005) *The World of Tattoo; An Illustrated History*. Amsterdam, KIT Publishers

Jones, C. P. (1957) "Stigma: Tattooing and Branding in Graeco–Roman Antiquity "

Andrea, P. (2004) ISBN 0-9650469-3-1   Kächelen,): *Tatau und Tattoo – Eine Epigraphik der Identitätskonstruktion.* Shaker Verlag, Aachen, ISBN 3-8322-2574-9.

Lombroso, Cesare (1896) "The Savage Origin of Tattooing",

Pang, Joey (2008) "Tattoo Art Expressions",

Raviv, Shaun (2006) "Marked for Life. Jews and Tattoos"

Stephens, B., Pratt, B. (1965)"Tattoos as fashion accessories" 1965Thomas,

Evelyn (1955)"African Tattoo Art", Willsboro Publishing

UNESCO, (2001) "Tattoo Folklore Preservation in Africa"

Xavier, A. Soto. C. (1964) "Mexican Tattoo Art", Publicadora Nacional de Artes

BOOKS BY THE SAME AUTHOR

"Gun Control, a Contradiction in Terms", by Julian Chitta

"American Marxism and Socialism", by Julian Chitta

"Texas Tales", by Julian Chitta

"IRS Secrets from the Nation's Cash Register", by Julian Chitta

"The Culture of Violence", by Julian Chitta

"Agenda 21", by Julian Chitta

"Lady Secret Agents", by Julian Chitta

"Soviet Military Intelligence Officer", by Julian Chitta

"Behold, I'm Jesus!", by Julian Chitta

"Accidental Scoops", by Julian Chitta

All these titles are available from amazon.com, in hard copy, or in Kindle format. Selected titles are also available as audio books, from audible.com, at affordable prices.

Copyright © 2010, 2014, 2018, by Julian Chitta. All Rights Reserved

www.ingramcontent.com/pod-product-compliance
Lightning Source LLC
Chambersburg PA
CBHW052334220526
45472CB00001B/414